THE POCKET GUIDE TO THE DSM-5-TR™ DIAGNOSTIC EXAM

T0200192

THE POCKET GUIDE TO THE DSM-5-TR™ DIAGNOSTIC EXAM

Abraham M. Nussbaum, M.D.

Chief Education Officer, Denver Health;
Associate Professor, Department of Psychiatry,
University of Colorado School of Medicine

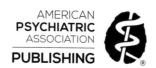

AMERICAN
PSYCHIATRIC
ASSOCIATION
PUBLISHING

Copyright © 2022 American Psychiatric Association Publishing

ALL RIGHTS RESERVED

First Edition

Manufactured in the United States of America on acid-free paper
26   25   24   23   22   5   4   3   2   1

American Psychiatric Association Publishing
800 Maine Avenue SW
Suite 900
Washington, DC 20024-2812
www.appi.org

Library of Congress Cataloging-in-Publication Data
Names: Nussbaum, Abraham M., author. | American Psychiatric Association Publishing, publisher.
Title: The pocket guide to the DSM-5-TR diagnostic exam / Abraham M. Nussbaum.
Other titles: Pocket guide to the Diagnostic and statistical manual of mental disorders-5-TR diagnostic exam
Description: First edition. | Washington, DC : American Psychiatric Association Publishing, [2022] | Includes bibliographical references and index.
Identifiers: LCCN 2021044464 | ISBN 9781615373574 (paperback ; alk. paper) | ISBN 9781615373581 (ebook)
Subjects: MESH: Diagnostic and statistical manual of mental disorders. 5th ed. | Mental Disorders—diagnosis | Interview, Psychological—methods | Physician-Patient Relations | Handbook
Classification: LCC RC469 | NLM WM 34 | DDC 616.89/075—dc23
LC record available at https://lccn.loc.gov/2021044464

British Library Cataloguing in Publication Data
A CIP record is available from the British Library.

Contents

Preface

You help others when you use the *Diagnostic and Statistical Manual of Mental Disorders*, Text Revision (DSM-5-TR; American Psychiatric Association 2022), an expansive catalog of mental illness, as a way to seek understanding of the people you meet as patients. For each illness, it provides diagnostic criteria and discusses the disorder from perspectives as diverse as culture, development, gender, genetics, law, and temperament. This book, *The Pocket Guide to the DSM-5-TR Diagnostic Exam*, is a pragmatic companion, a map for using DSM-5-TR when encountering another person for a diagnostic interview. This book is no replacement for either DSM-5-TR itself or psychiatric interview textbooks (see, e.g., MacKinnon et al. 2016; Shea 2017; Simpson and McDowell 2019; Sullivan 1954), but turns DSM-5-TR into a tool for an impactful diagnostic interview.

I often interview patients with students, trainees, and fellow practitioners, and I wrote this book so interviewers at all levels of experience could incorporate the structure of DSM-5-TR into their patient encounters. This guide follows the structure of DSM-5-TR. In the first section, I introduce the diagnostic interview. The first and second chapters address the goals of a diagnostic interview. The third chapter provides an efficient structure for learning the diagnostic interview. The fourth and fifth chapters describe how DSM-5-TR alters the interview. In the second section, I operationalize DSM-5-TR criteria for clinical practice. In the third section, I include diagnostic tools and additional information.

Taken as a whole, this book helps a clinician accurately diagnose a person in mental distress while establishing a therapeutic alliance, which remains the goal of any psychiatric encounter, even one as brief as a diagnostic interview.

Before beginning, a few words about language. In this book, because personhood precedes illness or consumption, I use the term *person* to describe the object of the initial diagnostic interview. When possible, I use gender-neutral terms for the person and the interviewer, but when doing so is grammatically awkward, I use the singular *they*. When speaking about a person who has entered psychiatric treatment after an initial interview, I use the term *patient* because it acknowledges the vulnerability of the person in treatment and the responsibilities assumed by mental health professionals when they care for patients (Radden and Sadler 2010). By using *patient*, I am not endorsing medical paternalism. Rather, I am emphasizing that the particular and protected relationships that develop in clinical encounters are better described as therapeutic relationships between a patient and clinician than as therapeutic contracts between a consumer and provider.

Acknowledgments

This book began out of my fumbling attempts to speak with people in mental distress, and is designed to improve those conversations, so I thank all the patients, students, and teachers I learned from along the way. Discretion prevents me from naming the patients. The passage of time impedes me from naming all the students. So I thank the teachers whose habits I try to emulate: Lossie Ortiz, Betsy Bolton, Andrew Ciferni, Stanley Hauerwas, Don Spencer, Sue Estroff, Amy Ursano, Gary Gala, David Moore, Julia Knerr, Karon Dawkins, Joel Yager, Eva Aagaard, Robert House, Vince Collins, Abby Lozano, Gareen Hamalian, and Michael Mizenko. Finally, I thank Melissa Musick, Melanie Rylander, and Helena Winston for reading (and improving) drafts of this book.

The revised version was primarily improved by dialogue with coauthors on related books, Robert J. Hilt, Warren Kinghorn, and Sophia Wang.

Disclosures

The author reports royalties from Yale University Press. Portions of this book are adapted from other books that the author previously co-authored with American Psychiatric Association Publishing.

Chapter 1

Introduction to the Diagnostic Interview

I no longer remember the author, but I never forgot her lesson. We shape each other with our questions. The author wrote about being out in public with her granddaughters. Strangers would approach her, unbidden, to tell her how sweet her granddaughters looked or how well they were dressed, and the author experienced grandmotherly pride. Then, one day, she encountered an older woman who, upon meeting the author's grandchildren, bent down and spoke directly to the girls, but not about their appearance. "What are you reading?" the stranger asked. A conversation between the stranger and the grandchildren ensued. The author was struck by the different ways that the stranger engaged the children: by asking after the books they favored rather than the clothes they wore, she was asking after how they understood their books instead of how they dressed their bodies. It is a different encounter for a young girl to be spoken *with* about what she is reading than to be spoken *of* regarding her appearance.

I am no grandmother, but her lesson surely applies to psychiatrists like me. When we ask questions of a person experiencing mental distress, we shape our experience of them. When my first question is about suicide or psychosis, I am asking a person to consider their mental distress.

From a practical perspective, this is apt because people encounter clinicians when they are experiencing mental distress.

When a person is experiencing mental distress, their first psychiatric encounter is often confusing or frightening. To a greater degree than in other areas of medicine, a person often has to overcome a series of obstacles before they are evaluated for mental distress (Radden and Sadler 2010). The obstacles can include access, expense, fear, and stigma, but once a person overcomes these particular hurdles, they deserve an encounter that acknowledges and names their suffering while initiating a working relationship. Although there are various ways to account for mental suffering, this book describes use of the most recent edition of the *Diagnostic and Statistical Manual of Mental Disorders* (DSM-5-TR; American Psychiatric Association 2022), the newest version of the common diagnostic language spoken by mental health professionals. DSM-5-TR has many perceptive critics (see, e.g., Allsopp et al. 2019; Caspi et al. 2020; Hayes and Hofmann 2020; Kendler 2014b; Kendler 2016; Raskin 2019). This book does not presume that DSM-5-TR is flawless or final, but that it is a shared way of organizing a psychiatric encounter into a diagnosis that contemporary professionals can pragmatically employ while seeking understanding of another person (Kinghorn 2011).

Understanding a person with mental illness who becomes a psychiatric patient is a remarkable challenge. People who become psychiatric patients often have overlapping vulnerabilities—including minority ethnicity, gender, language, race, religion, and sexual orientation—and fragmented experiences—including education, employment, housing, and relationships—that can be heightened by becoming a psychiatric patient. The psychiatrist Laura Roberts recently observed that a psychiatric patient's vulnerabilities "expand and augment the power of psychiatrists, psychologists, physicians, and mental health clinicians in subtle, complex, and often culturally determined ways" (Roberts 2016, p. 67). Clinicians need to be aware of the power they exercise in the clinical encounter so that their findings are something more than culturally predetermined.

Our challenge is that the findings of a psychiatric examination are neither as obvious nor as well understood as, for example, a subluxated shoulder, so mental health professionals need a common language like DSM-5-TR to describe these findings. Psychiatric findings are usually divided into *symptoms* (a person's subjective report of an abnormality) and *signs* (objective findings of an abnormality), but the most important thing is not the provenance of a finding but how a clinician uses clinical judgment to weigh symptoms and signs in the diagnostic process (King 1982). Although signs are generally considered more telling than symptoms, because they are observed, both are open to interpretation. When a person reports feeling tired, it can be a symptom of conditions as varied as anemia, anxiety, and apnea. When you observe a person crying, their tears may indicate glaucoma, grief, or grit trapped under a contact lens. A symptom like fatigue has little meaning independent of the person who is exhausted. A sign like tears matters because of the person whose cheek they fall upon.

Although many psychiatric symptoms and signs are particular to a specific mental illness, most are nonspecific—everyone has been fatigued, everyone has cried—and most people experiencing a psychiatric sign or symptom do not have a mental illness. Psychiatric symptoms and signs often exist in the borderlands between what is normal and what is pathological (Pierre 2010). Clearly, interpreting these symptoms and signs is difficult, and the risk of misdiagnosis is real, so you have an ethical responsibility to diagnose the suffering person before you as accurately as possible.

It is your responsibility to understand the relationships among the symptoms you elicit, the signs you observe, and their meaning for the person you meet. The effects can be profound, because although all illnesses threaten bodily integrity (Cassell 1991), mental disorders can compromise a person's ability to think, feel, and act. Because these faculties are centrally connected with a person's agency, sense of self, and identity (McHugh and Slavney 1998), mental disorders are often experienced as an existential threat. So when you see a person for the first time, remember that they may be internally asking something like, "What is wrong with me? Am I going crazy?" When you listen well to a person's report and identify the nature of the suffering, you can provide the relief that comes from giving a name to nameless fears.

The British internist Henry Cohen once wrote, "All diagnoses are provisional formulae designed for action" (Cohen 1943, p. 24). Diagnoses are provisional because they will be altered by further evidence. Diagnoses are designed because they are created by humans. Diagnoses are for action because they are intended to help a person effect a change in their health that they could not make without the clinician's diagnosis. When a clinician diagnoses a person, they inaugurate treatment, which makes a range of medically regulated experiences available to the patient. Cohen went on: "Diagnosis then implies an understanding of disease processes, their sites and their causes" (p. 25). Diagnosis is not a label, but a way of understanding. "Only by skill in observation, and interpretation in the light of knowledge and experience, only by exercising care and patience and by cultivating wisdom and judgment can be reached that most desirable of medical achievements—ability to diagnose disease" (p. 25). Diagnosis is an act of prudential judgment seeking understanding of another person.

A clinician should name suffering as accurately as they are able, and DSM-5-TR is a learned attempt to improve our clinical judgment as we characterize mental distress through the diagnoses of mental disorders.

DSM-5-TR improves the accuracy of psychiatric diagnoses by measuring the severity of a disorder, aligning diagnoses with the *International Statistical Classification of Diseases and Related Health Problems* (ICD) system, incorporating recent advances in the neurosciences, organizing diagnoses along developmental and lifespan pathways, increasing utility for forensic settings, reconceptualizing suicidal thoughts and behaviors, and deepening attention to culture, gender, and sex (American Psychiatric Association 2022). The edition revises the text of DSM-5, which was conceived by leaders of the American Psychiatric Association and other mental health groups, but ultimately crafted by many people organized into 6 study groups, 13 diagnostic work groups, and a task force of advocates, clinicians, and researchers (Regier et al. 2009). The resulting criteria were thrice made available online for public comment and field-tested for their reliability and validity (American Psychiatric Association 2013). DSM-5-TR extends their work by reviewing and revising the manual's text.

The signal advance of DSM-5-TR is the reengagement of social factors when diagnosing mental disorders. In this sense, it extends the DSM-5's introduction of "dimensions," or psychiatric symptoms that occur within and across specific disorders. Dimensions are discussed in Chapter 4, "Personalizing Diagnoses Through Dimensions," but in brief, they were introduced to reduce comorbidity and to begin moving toward a diagnostic system based on signs that indicate the dysfunction of neural circuits, rather than a diagnostic system based on symptoms. This marks a departure from previous DSM versions. DSM-5-TR extends this insight by adding other symptoms, chiefly suicidality, and by broadening the dimensions beyond symptoms, especially by increasing attention to how culture, gender, and sex affect a person's experience of mental health.

The authors of DSM began constructing diagnoses around the presence or absence of symptoms in the third edition (American Psychiatric Association 1980). This kind of diagnostic model is sometimes called a *categorical model,* because, based on the number of symptoms present, a person either does or does not have a mental illness that fits into a diagnostic category. Since DSM-III—the authors used Roman numerals for the first four editions but have switched to Arabic numerals to allow for the possibility of incremental updates (e.g., 5.1, 5.2)—the diagnostic criteria have included little mention of the cause of any particular mental disorder. This focus on symptoms over etiology is sometimes called "the atheoretic principle" (Wilson 1993). Focusing on the description rather than the cause of a disorder allowed mental health professionals who disagreed about the etiology of mental distress to work together. DSM-III proved useful for mental health practice and research, so subsequent revisions maintained the categorical model (Decker 2013). Its problems became more apparent over time, however. DSM began to look like a birding guide, in which external characteristics identified the species to which a bird belonged, irrespective of the cause of these characteristics (McHugh 2007), and, even worse, a birding guide whose fidelity during actual use in the proverbial field was unknown (First et al. 2014).

Richard Bentall, a British psychologist, once observed that because happy people are statistically rare, exhibit cognitive distortions like optimism, and experience a discrete cluster of symptoms, happiness is a mental disorder. Accordingly, Bentall proposed that people experiencing happiness be diagnosed with major affective disorder, pleasant type (Bentall 1992). Bentall was joking about the diagnosis but serious about his critique of a diagnostic system that was sometimes unable to distinguish the normal, but rare, from the pathological (Aragona 2009).

To respond to such concerns, the authors of DSM-5 added dimensional assessments, while refining the categorical model that most current clinicians know. Dimensional assessments allow clinicians to chart the presence of latent threats and vulnerabilities, which can be expressed or abated through the dynamic interaction between a person and their lived environment. (A person's obsessive traits may be, for example, beneficial in a health profession training program, and deleterious in a relationship, while being observable in both situations.) Because DSM-5-TR will be widely adopted, I wrote this book to guide both novice and seasoned interviewers as they conduct a DSM-5-TR diagnostic examination using both categorical and dimensional assessments. The book includes a practical discussion about initiating and developing a therapeutic alliance during a diagnostic examination (Chapter 2), spends several chapters observing how DSM-5-TR affects the diagnostic examination (Chapters 3–5), and continues with an operationalized version of DSM-5-TR for the purposes of conducting a diagnostic examination (Chapter 6). As we begin, it is useful to consider the work product of a diagnostic interview.

Disorders Instead of *Illnesses* or *Disease*

When you conduct a diagnostic interview, you generate a diagnosis, one of Cohen's "provisional formulae" for clinical actions. The diagnoses generated by a DSM-5-TR interview are called *disorders*, rather than *diseases* or *illnesses*. All three terms describe impairments of normal functioning, but the DSM system uses *disorders* to acknowledge the complex interplay of biological, social, cultural, and psychological factors involved in mental distress.

Physicians usually think in terms of diseases, which can be described as pathological abnormalities in the structure and function of body organs and systems. Patients usually present with *illnesses*, which are their experiences of pathological abnormalities or being sick. From a distance, diseases and illnesses may seem like the same experience viewed from the different perspectives of patient and physician. However, consider a condition such as hypertension, which is often identified incidentally, without any associated clinical findings. To the diagnosing physician, hypertension is a chronic disease of the vasculature that increases the risk of stroke and a heart attack, but patients often do not recognize themselves as being sick or as having an illness. Conversely, a patient may present as feeling quite ill and describe themselves as homesick, but physicians do not recognize this as a disease. Diseases and illnesses are often divergent experiences, rather than merely different perspectives, as anthropologists have repeatedly documented (Oberlander 2019).

An anthropologist can also tell you that illness experiences are culturally constructed: different conditions will be recognized as diseases or illnesses in different places and times. However, to be recognized as suffering from a disease or an illness, an individual requires some kind of diagnosis, often a diagnosis from a physician.

When a particular culture recognizes a person as suffering from a condition that alters one's place in the community, the person enters what American sociologist Talcott Parsons (1951) famously called the "sick role." Parsons observed that a person recognized as sick is exempted from normal social roles. Sick people do not have to perform their usual roles, but the degree of exemption from their social roles is relative to the nature and severity of their illness, as well as to their ages and cultural roles. To use contemporary examples, the child gets to stay home from school for mild fever and diarrhea, but the adult with back pain will receive disability only after experiencing years of refractory pain.

As part of the sick role, the sick person is usually not held responsible for their illness because sickness is believed to be beyond human control. So when a physician diagnoses a person with a sickness, the physician legitimizes the person's illness and admits them to the sick role (Parsons 1951). Admitting a person to a particular culture's sick role is part of what occurs when you diagnose a person's distress as a specific condition, and you need to remember that any diagnosis you assign to a person's distress has this cultural function.

Although all diagnoses have a cultural function, psychiatric diagnoses are especially complicated. Mental disorders result from biological, genetic, environmental, social, and psychological events and processes, and these etiological factors are involved to differing degrees in the development of different psychiatric diagnoses (Kendler 2012). Furthermore, because psychiatric diagnoses describe dysfunction in faculties believed to define one's personhood, they often constitute a threat to a person's sense of identity (Rüsch et al. 2005). Finally, the culture of clinicians and of medical facilities both shape the clinical encounter, altering what patients say and display and the outcomes they experience (Fiscella and Sanders 2016; Saini et al. 2017).

To recognize this complexity, the authors of DSM chose the term *disorder* to describe psychiatric diagnoses. *Disorder* can be broadly defined as a disturbance in physical or psychological functioning. The term is used elsewhere in medicine to describe genetic disorders and metabolic disorders. However, most diagnoses in medicine are called diseases rather than disorders, and naming psychiatric diagnoses as disorders reinforces a distinction between mental problems, *disorders,* and physical problems, *diseases* (Wallace 1994). We can see this when we consider that while a psychiatrist diagnoses a person with a "mental disorder," an internist does not diagnose a person with a "physical disease." Instead, an internist tersely diagnoses a person with a "disease," illustrating how our use of the adjective "mental" before "disorder" implicitly endorses a division between the body and the mind.

The authors of DSM-5-TR reduce this division by naming, whenever possible, the etiology of a mental disorder. They do so, for example, with several neurocognitive disorders (e.g., Lewy body, traumatic brain injury, vascular disease). However, the definition and limits of most categories of disorder remain broad. They range from illicit behaviors to particular pathological processes with well-characterized etiology, genetics, and prevalence. Therefore, the ambiguity about *what precisely a disorder is* remains.

Perhaps this is apt.

After all, diagnoses are an abstraction of a person's experiences and bear the marks of the era in which they were constructed and employed. Some diagnoses exist in one era and not another—hypertension, to return to our previous example, was not diagnosed in the 18th century because blood pressure could not consistently be measured. Some diagnoses serve one era's assumptions and not another's—as when psychiatric diagnoses were used to pathologize impoverished 19th-century Irish immigrants (Hirota 2017) and 20th-century Black activists (Metzl 2009) as part of racist, classist ideologies. Some diagnoses will be situated within psychiatry in one era and not in another. Some behaviors attendant to a seizure disorder, for example, can be attributed to epilepsy or to psychotic disorders (Sachdev 1998). Diagnoses serve cultural functions.

In this sense, using *disorder* to describe mental distress draws attention to how mental distress impairs a person's function, suggests the complex interplay of events that result in mental distress, and implicitly acknowledges the limits of our knowledge about the causes of mental distress. We do not know enough to be more precise. Instead, we can consider the ongoing use of *disorder* in our diagnostic systems as an opportunity for humility and a spur to further study. In the words of Ken Kendler, one of the most learned contemporary explorers of psychiatric diagnoses, "Tolerance for diversity and humility come with scientific maturity" (Kendler 2014a, p. 937).

The DSM-5-TR Definition of a Mental Disorder

The people you meet who have mental distress cannot simply wait for the precision that they and you desire—they deserve the best possible answers you can offer in the present moment. Cultural anthropologist Richard Shweder (2003) famously noted that anything observed from a single point of view is incomplete; incoherent when observed from all points of view at once; and empty if observed from no point of view at all. You have to take a particular point of view, but with the understanding that despite being necessary, the point of view you take is necessarily incomplete. It is far easier to criticize definitions of a mental disorder than it is to construct an accurate, precise, and useful definition.

According to the authors of DSM-5-TR, a mental disorder is "a syndrome characterized by clinically significant disturbance in an individual's cognition, emotion regulation, or behavior that reflects a dysfunction in the psychological, biological, or developmental processes underlying mental functioning." They distinguish a mental disorder from an "expectable or culturally approved response to a common stressor or loss, such as the death of a loved one." The authors caution, "Socially deviant behavior (e.g., political, religious, or sexual) and conflicts that are primarily between the individual and society are not mental disorders unless the deviance or conflict results from a dysfunction in the individual." This definition of a mental disorder, along with the authors' insistence that a diagnosis "have clinical utility" and "help clinicians to determine prognosis, treatment plans, and potential treatment outcomes for their patients" (American Psychiatric Association 2022), has several important implications for the diagnostic interview (Stein et al. 2010).

First, the definition characterizes a mental disorder as causing a clinically significant disturbance in a number of possible domains. This means that when you interview persons with mental distress, you need to explore the extent to which their distress significantly impairs their cognition, emotions, and behaviors. However, the definition does not characterize what constitutes a "significant" impairment. Without such precision, you need to define *impairment* with your patient based on how they functioned before the onset of the signs and symptoms with which they are presenting for evaluation. You might do this by asking the person to recall a time before the most recent onset of their distress and to describe the differences between their function at that point and in the present. Ideally, you will also obtain collateral information from people who know the person in multiple situations to help assess their premorbid ability and function. You may also want to use the World Health Organization Disability Assessment Schedule 2.0 (WHODAS 2.0), the disability assessment tool endorsed by the authors of DSM-5-TR (World Health Organization 2010), which is discussed in Chapter 12, "Selected DSM-5-TR Assessment Measures." Several other validated disability assessments are available, but whichever you use, you need to define *dysfunction* and *impairment*, along with their degree, individually for each person you evaluate.

Second, because the definition identifies dysfunction as occurring because of underlying disturbances in "the psychological, biological, or developmental processes underlying mental functioning," you need to assess all of these processes. The DSM-5-TR criteria offer clear guidance on how to elicit and organize symptoms of psychological processes, but provide less guidance for assessing biological and developmental processes. Because it is your responsibility to consider a person in full, you will need, at the least, to seek an understanding of the person's medical history and developmental stage. I briefly discuss ways to assess these processes in Chapter 3, "The 30-Minute Diagnostic Interview," and Chapter 8, "Six Questions to a Differential Diagnosis."

Third, the definition excludes dysfunction that is in some way expected. This can include responses to events such as the loss of an intimate relationship or employment—that is, events that induce mental distress in many people. The DSM-5-TR definition mentions "culturally approved" responses but does not define what constitutes either a culture or its approval, which further points to your need to assess the relationship between the symptoms you elicit in a diagnostic interview and their context in a person's life. Therefore, you might ask the person, or their family, friends, partners, and peers, if their response is consistent with the responses of their culture, because you need to explore the cultural context in which the person with mental distress presents.

Fourth, the definition simultaneously excludes dysfunction caused by a disagreement between a person and their broader culture. A person's thoughts and behaviors may clearly be in conflict with those of their intimates or with their culture. Conflict in and of itself is not evidence of a mental disorder. A person can disagree with the leaders of their country, disengage from their faith community, or dislike their siblings without having a mental disorder. For a diagnostic interview, establishing a person's cultural expectations and baseline behaviors is important, especially when you are interviewing a person whose age, gender, culture, experience, faith, language, or lifestyle is different from your own—in short, almost everyone you meet. You should ask a person what their distress means rather than make assumptions about its meaning.

Fifth, the definition includes an important caveat: a diagnosis must be clinically useful. This caveat helps further distinguish DSM-5-TR from a birding guide, because even if a person endorses all the symptoms of a particular disorder, if the disorder does not usefully inform that person's diagnosis, treatment, or prognosis, then the diagnosis is considered inappropriate. This requirement for clinical utility speaks to the pragmatic nature of DSM-5-TR, which is a diagnostic system designed to enable accurate and reliable communication of psychiatric findings, rather than to diagnose disorders simply for the sake of doing so.

The Questions Produced by a Diagnostic Interview

In reviewing the definition of a DSM-5-TR mental disorder, it becomes clear that the authors of DSM-5-TR left much undefined. This lack of definition necessitates, as happens so often in psychiatry, the exercise of practical wisdom (Radden and Sadler 2010). In the diagnostic interview, it means applying diagnostic categories to the irreducibly particular person before you. To define a mental disorder for the person before you, you need to seek a thorough understanding of the patient as a person. While a good diagnostic interview produces a diagnosis, it also generates questions you will need to ask as you seek understanding. These questions can relate to diagnosis, treatment, and prognosis.

At the conclusion of any diagnostic interview, you should generate a list of additional information you need for a more actionable diagnosis. This additional information can be as straightforward as collateral information from people who know your patient in other contexts, including reports from past psychiatrists, psychologists, therapists, counselors, primary care physicians, pastors, employers, coworkers, teachers, peers, friends, family, partners, and spouses. At times, you may wish to address particular areas of concern by administering additional diagnostic tests, such as physical or neurological examinations, or neuropsychological or personality tests. Before you administer additional tests, you should understand the strengths and limitations of each test and consider how a positive or a negative test result will change your therapeutic relationship. Finally, it is always useful to seek further understanding of a person's coping strategies and their understanding of the etiology and treatment of mental distress. People *present* with their distress, but *they are not* their distress. So ask after their strengths, their passions—about the activities that constitute their flourishing (VanderWeele 2020).

Although DSM-5-TR is not a treatment manual, the diagnostic interview is a time to consider whether and what treatment is indicated (cf. Hilt and Nussbaum 2016; Wang and Nussbaum 2017). With experience, you can initiate treatment in the interview by incorporating basic therapeutic techniques into your diagnostic interview. Many teachers recommend a classic text, *The Psychiatric Interview in Clinical Practice* (MacKinnon et al. 2016), to learn how to organize a psychiatric interview for the personality structure of your patient. If you feel presently unable to introduce therapeutic techniques into your diagnostic interview, you should at least begin mentally formulating the case and identifying resources keyed to the person's particular problems and strengths as you interview them. Ways to do so are discussed in subsequent chapters.

Finally, DSM-5-TR offers nothing in the way of prognosis to help a patient know what to expect of the treatment you recommend. You ought to offer reasonable hope to the person you interview. This hope should be informed by an evidence-based review of the scientific literature, your clinical wisdom, and your understanding of the person's premorbid functioning and of the available resources, but also by the possibility that the existing resources could be expanded through clinical advocacy. There are, after all, many kinds of clinical actions.

Conclusion

Critics of DSM-5-TR are concerned that it will be used as a psychiatric checklist rather than as a means for a comprehensive examination (see, e.g., McHugh and Slavney 2012). DSM-5-TR certainly can be received and misused that way. You can also employ it as one part of a comprehensive diagnostic interview that both characterizes the distress a person describes and helps in beginning to understand the person experiencing the distress. DSM-5-TR continues to rely on the experiences and symptoms reported by a person, but you can receive this as an implicit acknowledgment of the limits of the available knowledge about mental distress and an invitation to attend closely to each patient. In this fashion, your use of DSM-5-TR reflects your orientation toward the well-being of your patients, as well as your humility and willingness to revise your "provisional formulae" as you gain further insight and seek the ever-more fitting clinical action to which they aspire. In short, you can use a DSM-5-TR diagnosis both as an invitation to understand a person's mental distress and as the beginning of a conversation, rather than its conclusion, to create provisional formulas for clinical action.

Chapter 2

Alliance Building During a Diagnostic Interview

Every encounter with a person, even the first meeting, should be therapeutic. How can you accomplish this, even in a diagnostic interview? As discussed in Chapter 1, "Introduction to the Diagnostic Interview," accurately naming a person's mental distress is itself a response to a patient's suffering. A diagnosis initiates the therapeutic response to a person's distress and inaugurates a relationship in which you and your patient mutually commit to the patient's well-being. This relationship, called a *therapeutic alliance,* is the foundation of all psychiatric treatments and should be formed during a diagnostic interview.

When a patient and clinician mutually identify treatment goals and ally themselves in pursuit of those goals, they establish the alliance that mobilizes healing forces within the patient by psychological means. As the psychologist Edward Bordin wrote, in his seminal formulation, the therapeutic alliance includes "three features: an agreement on goals, an assignment of task or a series of tasks, and the development of bonds" (Bordin 1979, p. 25). The goal is the "why" of treatment, what the patient and clinician are working toward, whether it be recovery or remission. The task is the "what" of treatment, the activities that enable a patient to pursue health, whether they be thought records or titration schedules. The bond is the "how" of treatment, the kind of affective relationship that develops between clinician and patient, whether it be consulting or caretaking (Kinghorn and Nussbaum 2021). Your ability to form these alliances profoundly influences the efficacy of your work with the patient, as well as your satisfaction with and resilience in this work (Summers and Barber 2003).

Different therapeutic responses to a patient emphasize different aspects of the alliance (cognitive-behavioral therapy is, for example, more task-focused), but it is the strength of the alliance that consistently affects treatment outcomes. In a recent meta-analysis of hundreds of psychotherapy studies assessing the care of more than 30,000 patients from around the world, researchers found that developing a therapeutic alliance had a positive, medium effect size on treatment outcomes with both face-to-face and internet-based psychotherapies (Flückiger et al. 2018). In a smaller meta-analysis examining the role the therapeutic alliance plays in the medication treatment of persons with serious mental illness—that is, bipolar disorder, major depressive disorder, and schizophrenia—researchers found that when a clinician improves their alliances with patients, in either inpatient or outpatient settings, patients experience better treatment outcomes. Roughly, the same medication prescribed for the same condition produces about a 10% better patient outcome if it is prescribed within a positive therapeutic alliance (Totura et al. 2018).

Anyone who wants to know how and why the same treatment can be more effective within a therapeutic alliance should read Jerome and Julia Frank's classic *Persuasion and Healing: A Comparative Study of Psychotherapy* (Frank and Frank 1991). The Franks spent their careers asking why different forms of therapy—psychoanalysis, cognitive-behavioral therapy, group therapy, and Alcoholics Anonymous—as well as shamanistic encounters and religious faith can all effectively motivate change. The Franks observed that most aspects of a person cannot be changed because most people have a fairly fixed set of assumptions about themselves and the world. If these assumptions are fixed, why do people seek out mental health practitioners? According to the Franks, people have maladaptive assumptions about themselves and the world. These assumptions repeatedly fail, which is demoralizing. The Franks write that the "major sources of demoralization are the pathogenic meanings patients attribute to feelings and events in their lives. . . . Effective psychotherapies combat demoralization by persuading patients to transform these pathogenic meanings to ones that rekindle hope, enhance mastery, heighten self-esteem, and reintegrate patients with their groups" (Frank and Frank 1991, p. 52). Even during a diagnostic interview, you can identify maladaptive assumptions and the resulting demoralization. You can also rekindle hope.

The Franks found that all effective forms of therapy identify a socially sanctioned healer, a demoralized sufferer who seeks relief from the healer, and a circumscribed relationship in which they meet. To provide effective therapy, you must identify with a particular theory and have an appropriate confidence in it.

The Franks concluded that therapy is a kind of rhetoric in which you stimulate emotional arousal to transform the meaning of an event. That transformation occurs only if you offer the patient a conceptual framework for making sense of their maladaptive assumptions and the resulting demoralization. You can effectively invoke serotonin receptors or the superego, so long as the framework is compelling to the patient and to you. You can begin this process in the initial interview (Alarcón and Frank 2011).

Think about your own life: Did you ever work with a teacher or coach who helped you master a skill you could not learn on your own? How were you motivated? What was your relationship with the motivator? Now think about a teacher or coach for whom you underperformed. How were you discouraged? What was the nature of that relationship?

Your own goal should be to foster relationships that motivate people to make therapeutic changes in their lives, changes they could not initiate without the therapeutic relationship you share.

This is not to say that you need to mimic your favorite coach, teacher, or anyone else for that matter. During my own training, many of us went through a painful period in which we began talking earnestly in faux therapist voices. We would greet each other guardedly, fearful that expressing any emotion or personal thought would fatally betray our faults. The less confident residents (guilty!) bought tweed jackets and parroted our faculty. The more confident residents quickly moved beyond this stage and established their own styles. They showed me that a confident Texan, an assiduous Ohioan, and a mannered South Carolinian could all be effective if they could connect with their patients. Diverse approaches and styles can be therapeutic; you will become a better clinician as you develop your own style.

After all, if accurately applying the DSM-5-TR diagnostic criteria in all their specificity is the *science* of psychiatric interviewing, then the *art* is forming a therapeutic alliance. In an evidence-based and artful diagnostic interview, you conduct a form of rudimentary psychotherapy in which you instill hope and provide appropriate support to a demoralized patient. As you assess a patient, your goal should be to initiate therapy, because this helps reinforce the patient's intentionality, directing their thoughts toward health (Mundt and Backenstrass 2005). Here are a few evidence-based and artful ways to form a therapeutic alliance during a DSM-5-TR diagnostic interview.

Goals: The *Why* of Alliance Building in a Diagnostic Interview

When clinicians see patients, we often focus on what ails them, on their pathology. We ask after symptoms. We observe signs. We map them onto known disorders. We can build an alliance by mapping them onto specific, measurable treatment goals, as discussed in Chapter 10, "Mental Health Treatment Planning." Strive to instead leave the clinical encounter agreeing with the patient on *what matters most*, by asking yourself something like, "What are this patient's health goals, now and in the future?," and make sure you have a plan to prioritize the patient's goals (Zulman et al. 2020).

But remember: these goals are milestones along the way toward health, rather than health itself.

While we desire to know and name a patient's distress, the ultimate goal of a diagnostic interview is to encourage a patient's flourishing. The study of human flourishing has found evidence that cognitive exercises, behavioral changes, engagement in institutional and relational practices, and the addressing of psychological distress promote well-being (see, e.g., VanderWeele 2020). Seeking the well-being of the people we meet as patients is the ultimate *why* of the diagnostic interview.

Tasks: The *What* of Alliance Building in a Diagnostic Interview

A therapeutic alliance is also established by asking questions about the *what* of treatment, the tasks a person will undertake in pursuit of health. To do so, you need to establish a mutual framework for understanding the psychiatric signs and symptoms you elicit during a diagnostic interview. These framing questions simultaneously generate clinical information while building the therapeutic alliance.

There are many ways to do so, but I include two here. In the first instance, you build the alliance by asking about the patient's cultural experience of illness. In the second instance, you build the alliance by asking for an abbreviated version of their social history. Either method engages someone as a person before engaging them as a patient.

The psychiatrist and anthropologist Arthur Kleinman spent his career reflecting on what it means for people of different cultures to meet during times of illness. He found that physicians often assume they know what the meaning of an illness is for an ill person. When Kleinman and his colleagues asked about, rather than assumed, the meaning of an illness, they heard something quite distinct from what they expected. Based on these findings, Kleinman encouraged physicians to act like anthropologists and ask a person what their illness means, using these 10 questions adapted from Kleinman et al. (1978, p. 256):

1. What do you think caused your problem?
2. Why do you think it started when it did?
3. What do you think your sickness does to you?
4. How does it work?
5. How severe is your sickness?
6. Do you think it will have a short or long course?
7. What kind of treatment do you think you should receive?
8. What are the most important results you hope to receive from this treatment?
9. What are the chief problems your sickness has caused for you?
10. What do you fear most about your sickness?

By asking these questions, you begin understanding their mental distress and cultural account of their illness. You also build the alliance by exhibiting a sense of curiosity and humility about the patient and their particular culture.

If this approach seems too involved, one of my teachers, Joel Yager, recommends asking four simple social history questions:

1. Where do you live?
2. With whom do you live?
3. How do you spend your days?
4. How do you support yourself?

These four simple questions simultaneously gather data for the social history and implicitly assess the patient's psychosocial functioning. These neutral, open-ended questions invite reflection on the patient's material, social, economic, and communal existence. They provide a context for the symptoms you elicit later and at the same time build an alliance by implicitly addressing them as a person before you address their status as a patient.

The authors of DSM-5-TR implicitly endorse this approach by including two tools for assessing culture, the Outline for Cultural Formulation (OCF) and the Cultural Formulation Interview (CFI), and by increasing attention to culture throughout the text revision.

Now that you have established the framework in which a person understands psychiatric signs and symptoms, ask a patient something like, "What kinds of help do you need to address your problem?" Be open to considering the full varieties of help a clinician can provide: a diagnosis that names and explains a person's distress, a medical or psychological intervention that reduces or resolves a person's distress, a social or cultural intervention that responds to a person's distress, and more. Identify, with the patient, various types of assistance or "tasks" they are seeking.

Then, get specific about which kinds of help you can actually provide. Not every possible assistance could (or should!) be provided by a clinician. So ask a patient something like, "Which of those tasks should we work on together to improve your health?" Be candid about the help you can and cannot provide. You might, for example, prescribe a progressive exercise regimen, but are more likely to refer a patient to a fitness instructor than to teach a patient how to perform the necessary movements.

As you develop a shared sense of the tasks necessary to pursue heath, determining which will be pursued apart and which will be pursued together within the therapeutic relationship, you further build the alliance.

Bonds: The *How* of Alliance Building in a Diagnostic Interview

In their analysis of how therapeutic encounters work, the Franks found that "effectiveness is primarily a quality of the therapist, not of a particular technique" (Frank and Frank 1991, p. 166). If you are convinced that only one particular technique is useful, the Franks' viewpoint may be discouraging. However, it can also have a positive effect by encouraging you to cultivate your skills as a therapist and to figure out which approach you like best, because all therapies can be effective and all share the core attribute of forming therapeutic alliances. As you become better able to form therapeutic alliances, you will improve your ability to practice any therapy.

Your ability to form an alliance with any particular patient, however, will be shaped by a person's experiences before they even meet you. When you meet someone in the emergency department, they may have waited hours, even days, to see you, so the encounter may be terse and tense. When you meet a person in the office of their longtime family physician, they may be trusting and tranquil. But these behaviors cannot be anticipated for all individuals. People bring to your encounter both conscious and unconscious associations about the place where you meet and your role in that place. You cannot control those associations, but you can be aware of them. Before you meet a person for the first time, try to ascertain how they arrived at your meeting place, how long they waited to see you, and what they hope will result from your encounter.

As you approach a person for an interview, you can begin forming the alliance, before you even speak, by taking some practical steps. If you provide an environment in which people are safe enough to speak about intimate matters, you implicitly increase their trust in you. Ideally, the environment should include a comfortable chair for each of you, positioned so that you and your patient can make or avoid eye contact as necessary. This setup encourages conversation. Sitting with a patient has been shown to increase their perception of the time you spend with them (Johnson et al. 2008). In a recent study, even though sitting physicians spent an average of 24 fewer seconds with patients than standing physicians, patients perceived the sitting physicians as spending an additional 90 seconds with them (Swayden et al. 2012). You can bend time—or at least a patient's experience of it—by sitting with someone.

Because you never know how someone will respond to your presence, it is a good practice to sit closest to the exit in case you need to leave abruptly. Indeed, sometimes a person may be too agitated to tolerate sitting with you. Hospital-based clinicians are used to thinking of universal precautions, being aware of the possibility of infection in every human encounter. As a psychiatrist, I always counsel trainees that universal precautions include being aware of the possibility of violence in every human encounter. So, when meeting a person for the first time, no matter the reason, I counsel taking measures to ensure the safety of patients, practitioners, and staff. If staff members check a person into a room before you meet them, it can be helpful to ask the staff members about their sense of the patient's behaviors and emotional state to determine if it is safe to conduct the interview alone. (This has the added benefit of building your working alliance with other members of a treatment team.) Although it is easier to preserve the confidentiality of a person's interview if you interview a person alone, it is prudent to interview them with appropriate professional assistance if they are so upset that you fear for their safety or your own. If you will be accompanied during the interview, explain the purpose of your encounter to your companion before you meet the person or begin the interview.

Whether you approach the person with assistance or on your own, you can use nonverbal cues to build the alliance. Dress with care to signify your respect. Wearing any necessary personal protective equipment signifies your commitment to health and infection control. If you are meeting a person in a large clinical setting, wearing a badge with your name, picture, and title provides a visual assurance of your identity and role. Many interviewers have tissues or a glass of water available in case a person becomes tearful; providing small aids to a person in distress can be reassuring symbols of your care (Yager 1989). When you are engaging people through digital or remote means, it is similarly important to set the clinical stage by considering your nonverbal cues by modeling professional appearance and an inclusive visual environment, but it is additionally important to assure availability and interactivity (Tremain et al. 2020).

Whether remote or in the room, once you are ready to begin, you should initiate the conversation with a statement that advances the therapeutic alliance. An interviewer might simply say, "I am Dr. Chatterjee, your attending physician. I read your chart and would like to know more about you. What do you like to be called?" This brief statement communicates your name, your role, and your preparation for the meeting. It then invites the patient to identify themselves as they choose. An opening like this simultaneously indicates that you are prepared for your meeting but aware of the limits of your knowledge.

Then, set expectations about time and intent. An interviewer might say, "I would like to spend a half-hour developing an initial understanding of you and your mental health, including a diagnosis." By giving an amount of time and a purpose for the encounter, a clinician prepares a patient for what to expect. Pick a period of time equal to, or less than, the amount of available time, because it is better to overperform than underdeliver. Setting clear expectations reassures most people by reducing worry over the unknown. It is also a kind of test, to see how a person uses the time available to them: do they obsessively track the remaining time, dismiss it as insufficient, declare themselves undeserving of the time, or attempt to fill it entirely? Each informs your diagnosis.

Finally, ask the person a question specific to their presentation. An interviewer might say, "I would like to know what you hope to receive from mental health treatment," but should develop a specific question for each patient that encourages them to reflect upon their experiences.

Then, give the patient what the philosopher Simone Weil called the rarest and purest form of generosity: your undivided attention (Pétrement 1976).

The ideal patient will then present a coherent and comprehensive account of their current problem, its relationship to past experiences, a working diagnosis, and a treatment plan. That ideal is a fantasy, but you should listen for 2–3 minutes without interrupting as the patient tells their story, in whatever fashion they choose.

If you listen actively, you can further advance the therapeutic alliance, because active listening communicates respect for a patient and their concerns. As you listen, adopt a neutral but caring posture that communicates your attention and concern without betraying commitment to a particular interpretation of the patient's account. You are committed to the patient and their well-being, not to their interpretation of events. Avoid a premature rush to either judgment or solutions, both of which may seem like shortcuts to building an alliance but commit you to an initial interpretation that will inevitably be complicated by further information.

As you listen to a patient, it is common to hear what they are saying and, with experience, how they are saying it. You should eventually ascertain to whom the patient is speaking. In any conversation, people unconsciously assume role relationships. In a clinical encounter, a patient may receive you as a loving parent, as a cruel peer, or as an indifferent partner. A skilled therapist quickly ascertains how a patient conceptualizes the people they trust and distrust. In a good therapeutic alliance, you modulate your interview in response to a patient's needs.

This is a complicated skill, and learning it requires practice. A classic model for this skill is Otto Kernberg's (1984) *Severe Personality Disorders*. The entire book, especially the first two chapters, is important for anyone interested in considering how to understand role relationships during a diagnostic interview. Drawing on Kernberg's work, I recommend that as you interview a patient, you silently ask yourself these questions:

- Who is this patient addressing?
- How is this patient experiencing me?
- How is this patient portraying themself?
- How does this patient describe the personality of, and their relationship with, their mother, father, siblings, previous therapist, or other important caretakers or people in their lives?

Learning to reflect on how a patient perceives and relates to other people advances your understanding of them. This kind of reflection also deepens the therapeutic alliance. You can cultivate this habit—thinking about and with other people—even during a diagnostic interview.

As you actively listen, build the alliance by using nonverbal cues, such as head nodding, facial expressions, appropriate eye contact, and other signs of active listening (Robertson 2005). Expressing sympathy is appropriate, especially when a patient reports an event that causes them visible distress. Never express sympathy with statements like "I know what you are going through," because you want to maintain the focus on the patient. Instead, show empathy—which is both the cognitive act of recognizing someone in need and the affective act of sharing their suffering (Davies 2001)—through facial expressions and by providing reassurance when appropriate. If the person expresses fear that they are "doing it wrong," reassure them briefly: "You are doing fine" (Morrison and Muñoz 2009).

When you express concern, make it about a patient's well-being, not only about how they are adhering to treatment (Weiden 2007) or how well their symptoms and behaviors fit the criteria for a specific mental disorder. In a diagnostic interview, you can express concern about someone's well-being directly, by saying something like, "I hope you are okay," but it is especially helpful to express concern in a manner that simultaneously helps you better understand the patient. The statements that most profoundly build a therapeutic alliance are follow-up questions (Huang et al. 2017). So try something that expresses concern while seeking more details, like "I hear your concern and would like to know more about how it affects you and your relationships with other people."

Allowing a patient to tell their story, taking the time to discuss their concerns, respecting their feelings, and collaborating with a patient are all evidence-based techniques that build the alliance (Pinto et al. 2012).

In a diagnostic interview, you want to manifest empathy and warmth toward your patient through active listening by cultivating a style that is at once courteous, conversational, and comprehensive. As you do so, you form the affective bonds necessary for an alliance.

Conclusion

People do not seek your assistance to determine if their mental distress meets diagnostic criteria. The core of the diagnostic interview is not a checklist assessment of their psychiatric symptoms, but rather the formation of a therapeutic alliance, which involves learning to think *with* your patient. A therapeutic alliance is a relationship in which you and a patient in distress work together to reduce their distress and increase their sense of agency. In an effective diagnostic interview, you conduct a form of rudimentary psychotherapy in which you instill hope and provide support to a demoralized patient. The practical steps you take to form a therapeutic alliance improve the experience and outcomes of patient and clinician alike; the evidence for doing so and the strategies particular to categories of mental disorder are described elsewhere (Kinghorn and Nussbaum 2021).

Here, we conclude that developing the ability to form therapeutic alliances changes a clinician. A clinician becomes the kind of person who can aid a person in mental distress. So when the British psychiatrist Joanna Cannon recently reflected on her own training, she wrote:

> I learned that saving a life often has nothing to do with a scalpel or a defibrillator. I learned that lives are not just saved on the floor or an A&E department or in a surgical theatre. Lives are also saved in quiet corners of a ward. During a conversation in a garden. On a sofa in a TV room, when everyone else has left. Lives can be saved by spotting something lying hidden in a history. Lives can be saved by building up so much trust with a patient, they will still take a medication even if they don't believe they need it. Lives can be saved by listening to someone who has spent their entire life never being heard. (Cannon 2019, pp. 13–14)

Chapter 3

The 30-Minute Diagnostic Interview

If you are efficient and empathetic, you can elicit the essential psychiatric symptoms and personality traits of a person in 30 minutes. To do so, you must deliberately practice.

My own season of deliberate practice occurred while preparing for my oral board examinations. Even though I had seen hundreds of patients during the 4 years of psychiatry residency, I read a stack of interview books (e.g., Carlat 2005; MacKinnon et al. 2006; Morrison and Muñoz 2009; Shea 1998; Sullivan 1954; Zimmerman 1994) and adapted their advice into a timed outline for a 30-minute diagnostic examination. I practiced this exam 30 times until it became second nature, asked expert interviewers to observe me, learned from their constructive feedback, and passed my exams.

Since then, I have taught this version of the diagnostic examination to students, residents, and clinicians at all levels, modifying it along the way to account for DSM-5 and the growing science of how to build therapeutic alliances (Kinghorn and Nussbaum 2021). The resulting outline, provided below, is timed and includes both general guidance and italicized question prompts.

The outline is a guide, not an invitation to become a psychiatric robot who reads out screening questions at preordained intervals.

A robot moves abruptly from question to question, without transition or regard for the person before them. That style is what communication researchers call asking "full-switch questions." And they have found that when you shift quickly from one topic to another, you erode your alliance with a patient. Asking, "Are you suicidal? Are you hearing voices? Can you subtract 7 from 100?" in rapid succession demonstrates more attention to your need for information than to the specific person before you.

Rather, you should tailor the outline to the person presenting with distress, spending more or less time on a specific area based on their needs. A more organized patient may offer a concise history that you only need to clarify, whereas a patient displaying signs of mania or psychosis may be so disorganized that you will have to structure the interview. When you need to change the subject, use partial-switch questions—"I hear you are suicidal, but can you tell me how long you have been depressed?"—to preserve a human flow. Even better, you will build the alliance (and usually learn more) by asking as many follow-up questions, like "Can you tell me more?," as you can (Huang et al. 2017).

To tailor the interview, you must first learn how to construct it. While you are developing your own interview style, it helps to practice a formal version until it becomes a habit. I recommend practicing a timed version of this exam with patients from many backgrounds and with many presentations. The 30-minute diagnostic interview may seem forced at first, but it gradually becomes a habit and the underlying infrastructure for a conversational interview.

Outline of the 30-Minute Diagnostic Interview

The interview outline below includes headings that indicate the suggested time to allot for the following portion of the interview (boldface type), instructions to the interviewer (roman type), and statements that are questions for the interviewer to ask (italic type).

Minute 1

Introduce yourself to the person, including your role in their care. Ask how they would like to be addressed. Set expectations for how much time you will meet and what you will accomplish together. Then ask: *Why are you in psychiatric treatment?*

Minutes 2–4

Listen. A person's uninterrupted speech displays much of their mental status, guides your history taking, and builds the alliance. Although you may be tempted to interrupt or begin asking questions, with experience you will find that allowing the person to talk initially without interruptions gives you more information than the answers to your questions. Depending on the nature of the illness, some people will be unable to fill this time; their inability to do so also reveals valuable information regarding their mental status and distress. In cases where the person does not speak spontaneously, you may have to use prompts and proceed to the history of the present illness. Remember: the clinician who is silent at first is often heard afterward.

Minutes 5–12

History of present illness.   Your questions should follow the DSM-5-TR criteria, as operationalized in Chapter 6, "The DSM-5-TR Diagnostic Interview," and summarized in Chapter 7, "A Brief Version of DSM-5-TR." You should also focus on what has changed recently—the "why now?" of the presentation. As you do, you seek understanding of precipitating events by asking questions like: *When did your current distress begin? When was the last time you felt emotionally well? Can you identify any precipitating, perpetuating, or extenuating events? How have your thoughts and behaviors affected your ability to function with family, friends, and your community? How do you view your current level of functioning, and how is it different from what it was days, weeks, or months ago?*

Past psychiatric history.   *When did you first notice symptoms? When did you first seek treatment? Did you ever experience a full recovery? Have you ever been hospitalized? How many times? What was the reason for those hospitalizations, and how long were you hospitalized? Do you receive outpatient mental health treatment? Do you take medications for a mental illness? Which medicines have helped the most? Did you have any adverse effects to any medications? What was the reason for stopping prior medications? How long were you taking each medication, and how often did you take it? Do you know the name, strength, and number of doses per day of medicines you're currently taking, including over-the-counter and herbal medicines? Have you ever received injectable medications or electroconvulsive therapy?*

Safety.   Some clinicians feel uncomfortable asking safety questions, worrying they will upset people or even give them ideas about ways to hurt themselves or others. These fears are largely unfounded, and with practice a clinician finds these questions become easier to ask. They are always essential for an overall risk assessment. *Do you frequently think about hurting yourself? Have you ever attempted to kill yourself? How many attempts have you made? What did you do? What medical or psychiatric treatment did you receive after these attempts? Do you often have times when you become so upset that you make or even act upon verbal or physical threats to hurt other people, animals, or property? Have you ever been aggressive to people or animals, destroyed property, deceived other people, or stolen things?* (See "Disruptive, Impulse-Control, and Conduct Disorders," pp. 129–134, in Chapter 6.)

Minutes 13–17

Review of systems. The psychiatric review of systems is a brief overview of common psychiatric symptoms that you may not have elicited in the history of present illness portion of your interview. If a person answers affirmatively to the following questions, you should explore them further using the DSM-5-TR criteria, as modeled in Chapter 6.

MOOD. *Have you been feeling sad, empty, or irritable? Have you lost interest in, or do you get less pleasure from, the things you used to enjoy? Have there been times, lasting at least a few days, when you felt really "up" or irritable, and had a lot more energy than usual?* (See "Depressive Disorders," pp. 87–91, or "Bipolar and Related Disorders," pp. 83–87, in Chapter 6.)

PSYCHOSIS. *Have you seen visions or other things that other people did not see? Have you heard noises, sounds, or voices that other people did not hear? Do you ever feel like people are following you or trying to hurt you in some way? Have you ever felt that you had special powers, such as reading other people's minds? While watching television or listening to music, have you ever felt that it was referring to you?* (See "Schizophrenia Spectrum and Other Psychotic Disorders," pp. 79–82, in Chapter 6.)

ANXIETY. *During the past several months, have you frequently been worried about a number of things in your life? Is it hard for you to control or stop your worrying? Are there specific objects, places, or social situations that make you feel very anxious or fearful? A panic attack is a sudden surge of intense fear that comes on for no apparent reason, or in situations where you did not expect it to occur. Have you experienced recurrent panic attacks?"* (See "Anxiety Disorders," pp. 92–96, in Chapter 6.)

OBSESSIONS AND COMPULSIONS. *Do you frequently experience intrusive and unwanted images, thoughts, or urges? Are there any physical acts you feel like you have to do in order to avoid or reduce the distress associated with these images, thoughts, or urges?* (See "Obsessive-Compulsive and Related Disorders," pp. 96–99, in Chapter 6.)

TRAUMA. *What is the worst thing that has ever happened to you? Have you ever experienced or witnessed an event in which you were seriously injured or your life was in danger, or you thought you were going to be seriously injured or endangered? I am going to ask you a very personal question and if you are not comfortable answering, please let me know: Have you ever been physically, emotionally, or sexually abused?* (See "Trauma- and Stressor-Related Disorders," pp. 99–104, in Chapter 6.)

DISSOCIATION. *Everyone has trouble remembering things sometimes, but do you ever lose time, forget important details about yourself, or find evidence that you took part in events you cannot recall? Do you ever feel like people or places that are familiar to you are unreal, or that you are so detached from your body that it is like you are standing outside your body or watching yourself?* (See "Dissociative Disorders," pp. 104–106, in Chapter 6.)

SOMATIC CONCERNS. *Do you worry about your physical health more than most people? Do you get sick more often than most people?* (See "Somatic Symptom and Related Disorders," pp. 106–109, in Chapter 6.)

EATING AND FEEDING. *What do you think of your appearance? Do you ever restrict or avoid particular foods so much that it negatively affects your health or weight?* (See "Feeding and Eating Disorders," pp. 109–113, in Chapter 6.)

SLEEPING. *Is your sleep often inadequate or of poor quality? Alternatively, do you often experience excessive sleepiness? Do you frequently experience an irrepressible need to sleep or experience sudden lapses into sleep? Have you, or a sleeping partner, noticed any unusual behaviors while you sleep? Have you, or a sleeping partner, noticed that you stop breathing or gasp for air while sleeping?* (See "Sleep-Wake Disorders," pp. 114–121, in Chapter 6.)

SUBSTANCES AND OTHER ADDICTIONS. *How often do you drink alcohol? On an average day when you have at least one drink, how many total drinks do you end up having? Have you had any problems as a result of drinking? When you stop drinking, do you go through withdrawal?* Repeat for illicit and prescription drugs; begin by asking: *Have you ever experimented with drugs?* After asking about drugs, ask: *Do you bet, wager, or gamble in a way that interferes with your life?* (See "Substance-Related and Addictive Disorders," pp. 134–162, in Chapter 6.)

PERSONALITY.   *When anyone reflects on their life, they can identify patterns—characteristic thoughts, moods, and actions—that began when they were young and have since occurred in many personal and social situations. Thinking about your own life, can you identify patterns that have caused you significant problems with your friends or family, at work, or in another setting?* (See "Personality Disorders," pp. 169–179, in Chapter 6 or Chapter 13, "Dimensional Diagnosis of Personality Disorders.")

ELIMINATION.   *Have you repeatedly passed urine or feces onto your clothing, your bed, the floor, or another place where urine or feces are not usually deposited?* (See "Elimination Disorders," pp. 113–114, in Chapter 6.)

Minutes 18–23

Past medical history.   *Do you have any chronic medical problems? Have these illnesses affected you emotionally? Have you ever undergone surgery? Have you ever experienced a seizure or hit your head so hard that you lost consciousness? Do you take any medications for medical illness? Do you take any supplements, vitamins, or over-the-counter or herbal medicines regularly?*

Allergies.   *Are you allergic to any medications? Can you describe your allergy?*

Family history.   *Have any of your relatives ever had nervousness, a nervous breakdown, depression, mania, psychosis or schizophrenia, problems resulting from excessive drinking or drug abuse; made suicide attempts; or required psychiatric hospitalization? Have any of your first-degree relatives died by suicide?*

Developmental history.   *Do you know if your mother had any difficulties during her pregnancy or delivery? What were you like as a child? Did you have any problems during your early childhood? When did you reach puberty, and how did you feel about it?*

Social history.   *Did you have any behavioral or learning problems during your early childhood? When you started school, did you have trouble relating socially or keeping up academically with your classmates because of behavioral or learning problems? How far did you* *make it in school? Who lived in your home during your childhood? Was a religious faith part of your upbringing? Currently? How do you support yourself? How did you support yourself previously? What is the longest period of time you have stayed at one job? What jobs have you held in the last 5 years? Have you ever served in the military? How long and what rank did you achieve? What discharge did you receive? Have you ever been arrested? Jailed? Imprisoned? What do you like to do? How do you spend your time online? What do you like about yourself? What do your friends like about you? Do you have any confidants? Are you sexually active? Are there any particular urges, fantasies, or behaviors that repeatedly cause you to feel intensely aroused and worry you or other people?* (See "Paraphilic Disorders," pp. 179–181, in Chapter 6.) *Have you been less interested in sex than usual or experienced difficulties in sexual performance?* (See "Sexual Dysfunctions," pp. 121–127, in Chapter 6.) *Are you really uncomfortable with your birth-assigned gender?* (See "Gender Dysphoria," pp. 127–129, in Chapter 6.) *Do you feel safe in your current relationship? Are you, or have you ever been, married? Do you have any children? How old are they? Who is currently with the children?*

Minutes 24–28

Mental status examination (MSE).   You should have already observed or obtained most of the pertinent data. See Chapter 9, "A Mental Status Examination: With Essential Psychiatric Glossary," for a more detailed version of the MSE, which includes the following components:

- Appearance
- Behavior
- Speech
- Mood
- Affect
- Thought process
- Thought content
- Cognition and intellectual resources
- Insight/judgment: *What problems do you have? Are you sick in any way? What are your future plans?*

Mini-Cog: Screening for Cognitive Impairment in Older Adults. While many screening tools are available for cognitive impairment, the Mini-Cog comprises a three-item recall and a clock-drawing test and is an effective and efficient screening tool

(Tsoi et al. 2015). *I am going to say three words that I want you to repeat back to me now and try to remember. The words are: river, nation, finger. Please say them for me now.* Then say: *Now I would like you to draw a clock for me. First, put in all of the numbers where they go.* When the clock-drawing task is completed, say: *Now, set the hands to 10 past 11.* Finally, ask: *What were the three words I asked you to remember?* (Borson et al. 2003).

Minutes 29–30

Ask any follow-up questions. Thank the patient for their time and, if possible, begin discussing diagnosis and treatment.

Consider asking the following: *Have the questions I asked addressed your major concerns and problems? Is there anything important I missed or anything that I really should know about at this point to better understand what you are going through?*

Presenting the 30-Minute Diagnostic Interview

Just as it takes a habituated organization to complete this examination in 30 minutes, while altering its order and pace for each patient, it takes practice to present your findings. However, while you often have to supply the organization for a diagnostic interview, the presentation has an organization that you have likely learned in other contexts.

There are several reasons to practice the presentation as you practice your interview.

First, if you are a trainee, you will have to present a patient formally in order to earn board certification, as discussed in Chapter 11. Second, any clinician will find that when they formulate and present their account of a patient's mental distress, they clarify their own thoughts. A clinician's clarity will improve treatment plans and make written documentation more compelling to patients and other practitioners. When you successfully present a patient, you succinctly convey how well you understand them and their particular deficits and strengths. You also demonstrate your ability to organize the findings of your interview. To advance both skills, it is helpful to briefly consider how to present a diagnostic interview.

Gather your thoughts. Ask yourself if you can identify a central narrative from your interview. This is generally possible because most patients will present their distress as a story if you allow them to do so (Little 2005). For many patients, the story is revealed in the first words they speak. If you listen well, you will hear patterns in these stories; common narratives include acute distress following a dangerous experience, the progressive decline from a chronic illness, recurrence in the context of a stressful situation or an interruption in treatment, interpersonal troubles that are consistent with previous episodes in a patient's history, psychosocial events that demoralize a patient, or the development of behavioral patterns that cause distress. Clinical medicine is practical problem-solving through pattern recognition (Hunter 2005). If a narrative flows naturally from a patient's interview, organize your presentation around the narrative because it will help you remember your findings and will be more engaging to your audience. However, always include evidence that both supports and discredits the narrative.

When you speak, present the patient as a kind of story, introducing them by name, age, gender, and a chief complaint, preferably with a representative quote from the patient. (A friend of mine likes to add an illustrative detail here: the person's vocation or avocation, the language they prefer, or some other detail that is both clinically relevant and person-centered.) Follow with the history of their present illness, organized according to DSM-5-TR criteria, including pertinent information from the psychiatric review of systems. The middle portion of the presentation is the most straightforward—the past psychiatric history, the past medical history, family history, developmental history, and social history—but should be naturally connected to the central narrative of your presentation. So, for example, when presenting a patient experiencing a relapse during a chronic mental illness, the treatment history is comparatively more important than, say, the developmental history of a child making their initial presentation. In the last portion of the presentation, you should interpret the interview, describing the patient's mental status examination, along with your differential diagnosis, assessment, and plan. As discussed in Chapter 8, "Six Questions to a Differential Diagnosis," the differential diagnosis should include consideration of a patient's personality structure (with both deficits and strengths), substance use, cognitive ability or deficits, and other medical diagnoses that can mimic, alter, or otherwise complicate their treatment. You should always acknowledge your need for collateral, cross-sectional observation and serial examinations, as well as the limits of the history you obtained. Be sure to include predisposing biological, social, and psychological factors; current psychosocial stressors; and characteristic defenses in your formulation.

Be prepared to offer an integrated workup, treatment plan, and prognosis. One way to do so is by following an inverted pyramid, in which the most pressing concerns are addressed at the beginning.

1. Discuss any steps necessary to obtain or maintain **safety**. These should include the place where treatment should occur, the legal status of the patient, and what assistance they will need to maintain safety. In any presentation, safety precedes other concerns.
2. Address how the patient's **physical health** affects their treatment. In different settings, you might recommend a complete or focused physical examination, laboratory or imaging studies, referrals or consultations with other professionals, or nutritional or other treatments. Focus on the conditions influencing the patient's mental health.
3. Recommend any indicated **psychiatric treatment**, including psychoeducation, testing, therapeutic interventions, and medications. To the best of your ability, discuss the patient's past response to any medication; the cost of proposed medications; the known contraindications and interactions, along with any abuse potential; dose and dose titration; adverse effects and how you would ameliorate them; goal blood levels; the schedule of administration; whether the medications are best for short- or long-term use; and the cultural and legal consequences of treatment. Likewise, for any psychotherapy you recommend, describe the therapeutic problem, the recommended type of psychotherapy, the availability and affordability of therapy, the goal of therapy, and the motivation of the patient.
4. Address the patient's **social and cultural needs**. Discuss their strengths, living situation, significant relationships, employment, and community supports; the possibility of rehabilitative services; and any dependents. If you are concerned about the safety of a dependent, you should address it during the initial section of your formulation on safety.
5. Assess the patient's **prognosis** in relation to symptoms, treatment response, comorbid medical diagnoses, duration of illness, previous response to treatment, adherence to treat-

ment, availability and affordability of treatment, available social supports, and highest level of functioning.

As you present your findings, be appropriately self-critical. Admit any gaps or errors you recognize in your interview. Acknowledge your need for collateral and cross-sectional observations. Explain any deductions you made. Although the DSM-5-TR system is relatively more focused on symptoms than on signs, you should integrate a patient's signs into their symptoms and note any disjunction between signs and symptoms. Yet, be succinct. Present the entire case without interrupting yourself, but be prepared for your interlocutors to interrupt you. Your goal should be to simultaneously present the patient you interviewed and show your audience how you think about a person experiencing mental distress.

The practice is hard but rewarding. It will change you.

In the novel *Open City*, the protagonist is a psychiatry resident who reflects that "[a]t times, psychiatrists feel the absence of the neat solutions surgeons or pathologists enjoy, and it can be wearying to always have to find the mental preparation, the emotional focus, that is necessary for sitting with patients. The only thing, when I thought it all through, that enlivened the long hours I spent on call or in the office was the trust those patients had in me, their helplessness, their hope that I could help them get better" (Cole 2011, p. 44).

To realize that hope, practice.

Conclusion

When you conduct a diagnostic interview, you should listen actively. No matter how distracted or upset the patient is, you should always try to give them a few minutes to speak their own mind. As they speak, listen to the content and form of their statements. What are they saying? How are they saying it? What are they not saying? How do their statements match their appearance? Summarize and clarify their concern, then organize the exam as necessary, modulating the structure and language of the interview to fit the needs of the patient before you. Ask clear and succinct questions. If the patient is vague, seek precision. If they remain vague, explore why. Do not ask permission to change the subject, but use transition statements, such as *"I think I understand about this, but how about that?,"* to create partial-switch questions. Developing a supply of stock questions is helpful, which is why I advise using this structured interview until it becomes a habit through deliberate practice. Then you can use these questions to develop a conversational style for an interview in which a patient tells their story, you form an alliance with them, you gain insight into their thought process, and you gather the clinical data you need to make an accurate diagnosis. When you do so, you reduce the patient's alienation by making the strange more familiar.

Outline of the 15-Minute Diagnostic Interview

What if you only have 15 minutes? To gather the crucial information in 15 minutes requires a truly skilled interviewer. As you are developing this skill, remember that while you cannot generate a complete differential diagnosis and a comprehensive treatment plan in 15 minutes, you can seek the most likely diagnoses, identify a psychiatric emergency, and initiate treatment.

When meeting a patient for 15 minutes, I rely on five strategies:

1. Obtain background information before the interview. Selectively review any available records. Understand, if possible, why the patient is presenting today and with whom. Review any validated mental health screenings a patient and/or their caregiver completed prior to the visit. These screenings can give an idea of where to initially direct diagnostic questions.
2. Observe the patient's functional status during the interview. If possible, walk your patient to an examination room. This simple courtesy gives you an opportunity to observe how a patient dresses, greets a stranger, ambulates, and navigates a novel space.
3. Determine whether a patient's functional status matches their current level of social support and care. Learning how well a patient's psychosocial needs and their currently available resources fit together is a critical first step in a treatment plan.
4. Ask about safety. Briefly assess harm to self, harm to others, and substance use.

5. Ask about treatment choices. Offer options during treatment planning sessions: medications, psychotherapy, and psychosocial changes. By asking which treatments your patient will accept, you build the alliance.

Minute 0

Review the screening responses before meeting the patient. Formulate in your mind what areas you want to focus on and how you intend to structure your interview.

Minute 1

Introduce yourself and explain the length and purpose of today's interview.

Minutes 2–4

Start with a general statement such as "Tell me what brought you here" or a more specific question tied to the screening materials, such as "Tell me more about the depressive symptoms you have had recently." Listen for at least a minute. Allow a patient to narrate the history of their present illness rather than asking a list of closed-ended questions. Get a sense of how well the patient can organize their history, how long they have been experiencing these symptoms, and how they affect their daily routine.

Minutes 5–10

Perform a psychiatric review of systems and a brief cognitive screening that includes orientation and three-item delayed recall. If not possible, collect collateral information from the patient's caregiver(s).

Minutes 11–12

Collect past psychiatric history and screen for red flags such as suicide, abuse, and heavy substance use that will require you to refer your patient for further treatment, such as mental health or social work. For the psychiatric history, determine if or how long the person has been in mental health treatment; if they have been psychiatrically hospitalized; and if there have been any suicide or homicide attempts and, if so, the lethality of those attempts. For the psychotropic history, you primarily need to know which medications the patient has tried and had strongly positive or negative experiences with, if they are taking any medications from which they could withdraw, and whether they have ever taken a mood stabilizer and/or antipsychotic. You can accelerate this process by having them review a list of psychotropics beforehand to check which ones have been previously prescribed.

Minutes 13–15

By the end of the interview, you should know which of the three categories your patient fits in: 1) obtain further information and/or treat in primary care, 2) refer to mental health for further treatment, and 3) in very rare circumstances, make referral to emergency psychiatric services. Finally, you should share an initial treatment plan with the patient.

Chapter 4

Personalizing Diagnoses Through Dimensions

Have you ever met a patient with major depressive disorder who has experienced panic attacks? I meet them weekly, but panic attacks are not part of the diagnostic criteria for major depressive disorder, even though people with depression often seek clinical assistance for panic.

Have you ever struggled to decide how impaired a patient is by their schizophrenia? Some people with schizophrenia are profoundly disabled, some are high-functioning, and most people with schizophrenia live somewhere in between.

Have you ever met an anxious adolescent but been unsure how to efficiently determine if their anxiety was pathological? Most anxious adolescents will enter care in general medical practices, where few clinicians have extensive mental health training.

DSM-5-TR addresses these kinds of situations by incorporating a dimensional approach to psychiatric symptoms. These dimensions are used to measure symptoms in three ways in DSM-5-TR.

First, dimensions provide a way to acknowledge psychiatric symptoms that are not part of the diagnostic criteria of a patient's primary mental disorder. For example, if you treat a patient with major depressive disorder who also experiences panic attacks, you can add with panic attack as a specifier to the diagnosis.

Second, dimensions allow psychiatrists to measure the magnitude of a symptom. For example, DSM-5-TR includes Clinician-Rated Dimensions of Psychosis Symptom Severity, which consist of 8 domains rated on a 5-point scale for their severity, rather than just their presence or absence (see Chapter 12, "Selected DSM-5-TR Assessment Measures, pp. 225–230).

Third, dimensions provide a way to screen for mental disorders in general clinical populations. For example, before evaluating an adolescent, a pediatrician could ask the patient to complete the DSM-5-TR Self-Rated Level 1 Cross-Cutting Symptom Measure, which is available in DSM-5-TR (Section III), as well as online at www.psychiatry.org/dsm5, and is discussed briefly in Chapter 12, "Selected DSM-5-TR Assessment Measures." If the pediatrician went over the results with the adolescent and a generalized anxiety disorder was suspected, the pediatrician could refer the adolescent to a child and adolescent psychiatrist, who could ask the patient to complete an adolescent-specific assessment tool for anxiety disorders, called PROMIS Emotional Distress–Anxiety (available at www.psychiatry.org/dsm5), which assesses how frequently the patient experiences symptoms of anxiety. A child and adolescent psychiatrist could subsequently ask the patient to complete the PROMIS Emotional Distress–Anxiety assessment before each encounter so an interviewer could chart the patient's progress.

According to the architects of DSM-5-TR, the introduction of dimensions is their most important advance (Regier 2007). Why? Insightful critics have previously noted that the DSM diagnostic system could not always distinguish normality from pathology and one mental disorder from another (Kendell and Jablensky 2003). The architects of DSM-5-TR addressed these concerns by incorporating dimensions into their otherwise categorical diagnostic system.

Consider the examples from above.

In the instance of a panic-ridden patient with major depressive disorder, the use of dimensions allows you to identify their problem without adding an additional diagnosis. This distinguishes a patient with depression who is experiencing panic problems from a patient with both panic disorder and major depressive disorder.

In the instance of a patient with schizophrenia, the use of dimensions allows a clinician to assess the severity of the patient's disorder, thus better distinguishing normality from pathology, and charting his progress. In a strictly categorical system, a clinician determines only whether or not a person has a mental disorder. By adding dimensions, a clinician can grade the severity of a disorder as well as the particular symptoms that are most concerning to the patient, rather than simply declaring a patient does or does not have a disorder.

In the instance of the anxious adolescent, the use of dimensions leads to screening tools that supplement the diagnostic armamentarium of primary care providers and mental health practitioners alike.

How does the use of dimensions affect the diagnostic exam? The first implication is that you must screen for a wide range of psychopathology, because you cannot measure what you do not assess. The second implication is that you can record the symptoms you elicit and measure their severity. As you do so, keep in mind that dimensions supplement but do not replace the categories established in earlier DSM versions, as will be evident in the remainder of this chapter, which discusses some of the ways dimensions are (and are not) used in DSM-5-TR.

Severity Ratings

DSM-5-TR provides severity rating scales for many disorders. Most of these scales are specific to a particular disorder, and many include a narrative description to indicate that a particular disorder is mild, moderate, or severe. For some diagnoses, such as alcohol use disorder, severity depends on the number of criteria endorsed by a patient. In other instances, severity is measured by the degree to which a patient requires support, as in autism spectrum disorder. Where appropriate, the severity ratings refer to specific measurements external to the mental status examination. For example, you assess the severity of anorexia nervosa by describing a patient's body mass index. In short, the various severity scales are designed to help you go beyond diagnostic categories to focus on the particular patient you are evaluating.

The most groundbreaking of these tools is the Level of Personality Functioning Scale. This tool is discussed in Chapter 5, "Key Changes in DSM-5-TR," and in Chapter 13, "Dimensional Diagnosis of Personality Disorders," but here I want to observe that it allows you to assess a wide range of personality traits, so that you can distinguish between, for example, the antagonism expressed by a person with antisocial personality disorder and that expressed by someone with narcissistic personality disorder. In a categorical model, having, say, narcissistic personality disorder is a yes-or-no question, which encourages a stigmatization of people with personality disorders. Instead of saying someone has narcissistic personality disorder, we often say that someone is a narcissist. In a dimensional model, a clinician can express the various traits of personality disorders that a person has, the different degrees of severity of those traits, and how those traits can change over time (Newton-Howes et al. 2015). A dimensional model also offers an effective definition of mental health within DSM for the first time, with Level 0 (little or no impairment) on both the Self and Interpersonal scales implicitly indicating mental health.

The Level of Personality Functioning Scale was part of a proposed reconceptualization of personality disorders. This reconceptualization, discussed in Chapter 5, is included among DSM-5-TR's "Emerging Measures and Models" and has demonstrated its clinical utility (e.g., Barroilhet et al. 2020) and predictive power for clinical outcomes (Milinkovic and Tiliopoulos 2020) and relationship satisfaction (e.g., Ingram and South 2021). As this title suggests, if you familiarize yourself with the model described in Chapter 13, you will appreciate how a fully dimensional diagnostic system works. For now, DSM-5-TR uses dimensions in a more circumspect fashion.

Screening Tools

Most people will first seek help for mental distress from someone they already know. Within medicine, this will usually be a physician, nurse, or other professional who has typically not received specialized mental health training. Indeed, most mental health care occurs in the offices of primary care clinicians.

To address the gap between the mental health training that these clinicians possess and the volume of mental health care they provide, DSM-5-TR provides dimensional screening tools modeled on general medicine's review of systems. These brief, easy-to-read tools can be completed before a clinical encounter by the patient or someone who knows them well. Each tool has a series of short questions about recent symptoms; for example, "Have you been feeling more irritated, grouchy, or angry than usual?" These screening questions assess core symptoms for the major diagnoses. For each symptom statement, a patient will assess how much this bothered them using a five-point scale: none (1), slight (2), mild (3), moderate (4), or severe (5). Each tool is designed to be easily scored. If a patient reports a clinically significant problem in any domain, you should consider a more detailed assessment tool available from www.psychiatry.org/dsm5.

As this example suggests, DSM-5-TR includes a hierarchy of screening tools and dimensional assessments. The initial assessment, the Level 1 Cross-Cutting Symptom Measure, is the screening tool described in the previous paragraph, and it is completed by the person seeking assessment, before an initial evaluation, or by the parent or guardian of a child. The adult version includes 23 questions assessing 13 domains of psychiatric symptoms. The child version includes 25 questions assessing

12 domains. For most, but not all, of the symptom domains screened for in the Level 1 Cross-Cutting Symptom Measure, there are separate Level 2 Cross-Cutting Symptom Measures for specific areas of concern like anxiety. When Level 1 and 2 assessments are used, they help an interviewer identify and address the presenting problems.

Once a person enters treatment as a patient, how do you measure their response and progress toward recovery? DSM-5-TR encourages you to use these Level 2 Cross-Cutting Symptom Measures at your first evaluation of a patient in part so you can establish their baseline, and asks you then to revisit that assessment periodically to assess their progress. These measures assess dimensions (rather than diagnoses) that cut across diagnostic categories. These assessments allow you, for example, to track the depressive symptoms of a patient with schizophrenia in addition to their psychotic symptoms. Systematic use of these cross-cutting assessments will alert you to significant changes in a patient's symptomatology, will provide measurable outcomes for treatment plans, and, in aggregate, alert researchers to lacunae in the current diagnostic system and suggest new treatment strategies (see, e.g., Chekroud et al. 2017).

Cultural-Related Diagnostic Issues and Assessments

Culture develops out of folk and professional traditions; an indigenous community and a medical society both have a culture, a set of arts and customs, which they have cultivated from their shared life.

The authors of DSM-5-TR renewed attention to the ways culture affects diagnosis throughout the manual, often implicitly observing the ways in which folk and professional traditions interact. So, for example, in their discussion of pica, the authors noted that "[i]n some populations, the eating of earth or other seemingly nonnutritive substances is believed to be of spiritual, medicinal, or other social value, or may be a culturally supported or socially normative practice. Such behavior does not warrant a diagnosis of pica....Pica behavior may be prevalent in some cultural groups, but it should not be assumed to be socially normative without further evaluation" (American Psychiatric Association 2022, pp. 372–373).

In this statement, the authors navigate between normalizing and pathologizing behavior. They draw an interviewer's attention to the ways that the same behavior can be a cultural act and a medical symptom. Even more, they invite interviewers to further evaluate, to engage a patient further to understand the meaning of their experience. To help a clinician do so, the authors of DSM-5-TR have revised the "Culture-Related Diagnostic Issues" sections throughout the manual, updating their review of the data and their counsel to clinicians, while attending to the ways culture and psychiatric diagnosis have enabled racism and discrimination.

They have also included a glossary, an alphabetized catalogue, of cultural concepts of distress. The glossary briefly describes several conditions: *ataque de nervios* (intense emotional response among Latinx), *dhat* syndrome (anxiety and distress about semen loss among South Asian men), *hikikomori* (protracted social withdrawal observed in Japan), *khyâl cap* (catastrophic cognitions that a wind-like substance may arise in the body that is experienced as anxious distress among people from Cambodia), *kufungisia* (a range of psychopathology believed to result from worry among the Shona of Zimbabwe), *maladi dyab* (a social malice mediated through sorcerers and causing a wide range of distress experienced in Haitian communities), *nervios* (a vulnerability to stress resulting in a distressing experiences among Latinx), *shenjing shuairo* (a syndrome of weakness that brings Western and Chinese idioms), *susto* (symptoms experienced by some Latinx in which the soul is experienced as leaving the body in response to a frightening event), and *taijin kyofusho* (anxiety and avoidance of interpersonal encounters because of negative self-perception among people in Japan).

The glossary allows a clinician to observe the ways mental and physical symptoms overlap in folk and professional explanatory models, while providing references for clinicians interested in learning more about these experiences as they seek understanding of their patients.

As I discuss in Chapter 1, "Introduction to the Diagnostic Interview," distress, disease, and illness are all profoundly shaped by cultural forces. As recommended in Chapter 2, "Alliance Building During a Diagnostic Interview," asking about a patient's cultural understanding of sickness and health is an effective and efficient way to build a therapeutic alliance while gathering pertinent information (Aggarwal et al. 2020a). A clinician who performs a cultural assessment is also better able to identify and understand a patient's concerns, correctly diagnose their distress, receive additional information, personalize the diagnosis, and guide scientific discovery (Lewis-Fernández et al. 2016).

To use this cultural information in a diagnostic interview, it is beneficial to first define three types of cultural concepts. In Section III of DSM-5-TR, in "Culture and Psychiatric Diagnosis," the authors discuss cultural syndromes, cultural idioms of distress, and cultural explanations of perceived causes. A *cultural syndrome* is a group of clustered psychiatric symptoms specific to a particular culture or community. The syndrome provides a coherent pattern for experiences. A classic example is *ataque de nervios,* a syndrome of mental distress characterized by the sudden onset of intense fear, often experienced physically as a sensation of heat rising in the chest, that may result in aggressive or suicidal behavior (Lewis-Fernández et al. 2010). The syndrome is often associated with familial distress in Latinx communities across DSM-5-TR diagnostic categories (Lizardi et al. 2009). A *cultural idiom of distress* is a collective, shared way of expressing distress outside of a specific syndrome or symptom, say, "nerves" instead of *ataque de nervious* or generalized anxiety disorder. Finally, a *cultural explanation of perceived cause* provides an explanatory model of why mental distress or illness occurs, and the cultural explanation can be folk or professional, as both indigenous communities and medical societies constitute a culture (American Psychiatric Association 2022).

The Cultural Formulation Interview (CFI) is a semistructured tool, updated for DSM-5-TR, to assess the influence of culture in a particular patient's experience of distress. The CFI can be used at any time during a diagnostic interview, but the DSM-5-TR authors suggest using it when you are struggling to reach a diagnosis because of cultural differences between you and a patient, when you are uncertain if diagnostic criteria map onto a cultural concept, when you are laboring to assess the dimensional severity of a diagnosis, when you and a patient have divergent understandings of treatment, when you and a patient disagree on treatment, when a patient may mistrust health services because of a collective traumatic experience, or when a patient is disengaged during an interview (American Psychiatric Association 2022).

Over the last decade, the use of the CFI has been studied in Canada, Kenya, Mexico, the Netherlands, Peru, and the United States (Jarvis et al. 2020). With trainees, researchers have found that undertaking even a single hour of CFI training can increase a clinician's cultural competence (Mills et al. 2016), and CFI training can be delivered through online curricula (Aggarwal et al. 2018). The CFI can be the foundation of a culturally competent clinical service (Díaz et al. 2017), including forensics services (Aggarwal et al. 2020b).

You should not limit its use to situations in which you perceive the patient as culturally different from yourself. You can use the CFI profitably in any setting because "cultural" accounts of why people get ill and why people return to health occur in all communities. A person whom you believe to share your own cultural account of illness and health often has a very different understanding of why people become ill and how they can become well. Finally, the CFI is the most patient-centered portion of DSM-5-TR, and using it particularizes the diagnostic process. The CFI is not a scored system of symptoms but a series of prompts to help you assess how a patient understands his distress, its etiology, its treatment, and prognosis. I include an operationalized version of the CFI in Chapter 12 of this book, but additional information is available in DSM-5-TR itself. Online, at www.psychiatry.org/dsm5, you can find alternative versions of the CFI and supplementary modules.

Sex- and Gender-Related Diagnostic Issues

Previous editions of the DSM have famously excluded sexual minorities (cf. Nussbaum 2019). Less famously, previous editions incorporated multiple accounts of gender and sex without synchronizing them between diagnostic categories like gender dysphorias and sexual dysfunctions. DSM-5-TR addresses both by including in the text for each disorder, where applicable, a section on sex- and gender-related diagnostic issues.

So, in the text for posttraumatic stress disorder, the authors characterize the prevalence of PTSD by gender—8%–11% of women and 4.1%–5.4% in the United States—and observe that the difference is likely due to differences in interpersonal violence, emotional processing of trauma, and reproductive hormones between women and men.

DSM-5-TR uses gender differences—between women and men, boys and girls—because much of our information on psychiatric literature is based on these gender differences. Gender, within the manual, "is a result of reproductive organs as well as an individual's self-representation." When possible, as in pregnancy or menopause, the authors refer to sex differences, as male and female, and observe that they can cross diagnostic categories. So a specifier like "with peripartum onset" can apply to a brief psychotic disorder, or a depressive, hypomanic, or manic episode.

The authors have included, when available, information on both gender and sex. Throughout the text, the authors have worked to remove bias against sexual minorities and to understand gender and sex as resulting from the interplay of biological, cultural, and psychological factors.

Associations With Suicidal Thoughts or Behavior

We live in an era where life expectancy is decreasing, which leading researchers have attributed to a rise in the diseases of despair: mental illness, substance abuse, and suicide (Case and Deaton 2020)). The DSM has long included formal diagnostic criteria for mental illness and substance abuse but does not have a specific diagnosis for suicide, a leading cause of death. DSM-5-TR addresses suicide so thoughtfully, across so many conditions, that it functions as a kind of dimension within the manual. First, the text includes sections labeled "Association With Suicidal Thoughts or Behavior" that assess the available literature. So, for example, in the text for alcohol use disorder, DSM-5-TR draws clinicians' attention to the sevenfold increase in suicide attempts associated with the acute use of alcohol. These sections alert clinicians and help them to stratify risk so that they can intervene to prevent suicide.

Second, DSM-5-TR conceptualizes suicide as bidirectional. For example, in the text for insomnia disorder, the authors write that in a study of college students, 31.3% with sleep problems had suicidal thoughts, but 82.7% of individuals with suicidal thoughts experienced sleep problems. Being suicidal increases your risk of having a mental disorder; having a mental disorder increases your risk of being suicidal.

Third, DSM-5-TR updates the text for several related diagnoses for further study. Nonsuicidal self-injury disorder, characterized by a patient's intentional and repetitive inflection of minor to moderate painful injuries to the body's surface without suicidal intent, is a common clinical presentation, typically beginning in adolescence, and the activity often declines as people mature into adulthood. The diagnosis, while not included in the main text, is clinically useful, and a reminder that the DSM is a manual, rather than a kind of psychiatric scripture, updated to fit cultural contexts and clinical needs like today's various ways of self-harm and suicide that reinforce the metaphorical diseases of despair.

Conclusion

By introducing dimensions, the authors of DSM-5-TR are trying to increase the accuracy of current diagnoses, reduce the number of diagnoses ascribed to each patient, and account for the dynamic nature of diagnostic "categories" over a patient's life. They hope the clinical use of dimensions will identify relationships between disorders that were separated in strictly categorical diagnostic systems, such as DSM-IV. For example, although major depressive disorder and alcohol use disorder are known to be associated with each other, the precise nature of their association is unclear. To return to the situation with which this chapter began, the careful use of dimensions may help identify a subset of people whose depression is etiologically connected to their panic in a previously unknown fashion. In this way, a dimensional diagnostic system could spur research by identifying unknown connections or by explaining associations that are not yet understood.

The authors of DSM-5-TR introduced dimensions in a subtle fashion, chiefly for screening tools and rating systems. They piloted, but did not adopt, dimensional approaches to personality disorders. Dimensions remain the future of psychiatric diagnostic systems. At present, they have concluded that while dimensional measures increase diagnostic reliability and clinical communication, they are not sufficiently operationalized for everyday clinical use.

So, for now, most diagnoses will occur in categorical models. As I continue to use categorical models in my practice, I like to remember words of the poet Wallace Stevens:

> Description is revelation. It is not
> The thing described, nor false facsimile.
>
> It is an artificial thing that exists,
> In its own seeming, plainly visible, . . .

Categories are useful description, artificial revelations that exist as the result of the diagnostic process. But as we seek fuller understandings of our patients, we can all benefit from incorporating more dimensional assessements into our clinical encounters (e.g. Caspi and Moffitt 2018; Grisanzio et al. 2018). If you look at Chapter 14, "Alternative Diagnostic Systems and Rating Scales," you can see that the concept of dimensions has support from both psychoanalysts and neuroscientists. Practitioners can move toward that future today by employing DSM-5-TR's dimensional tools in clinical practice, as we seek "the thing described" by bettering our "artificial thing."

Chapter 5

Key Changes in DSM-5-TR

DSM-5-TR bridges the current diagnostic system, which is based on symptom categories, and a future diagnostic system based on disturbances in specific, interconnected circuits of the brain (Kupfer and Regier 2011). The essential supports in this bridge are the *dimensions*, which crisscross existing diagnostic categories, as discussed in Chapter 4, "Personalizing Diagnoses Through Dimensions." Clinicians also need to know about how the bridge itself, DSM-5-TR, is changing. The authors of DSM-5-TR drew upon the work of hundreds of clinicians and researchers to refine the diagnostic criteria for several diagnoses, add a diagnosis and a condition that may be a focus of clinical attention, change the names of a few diagnoses, and completely refine the text, all of which is reflected in Chapter 6, "The DSM-5-TR Diagnostic Interview." In this chapter, I present four case examples involving common diagnoses to display how the changes in DSM-5-TR alter the diagnostic interview. In the final section of this chapter, I describe how DSM-5-TR reorders disorders for development and temperament.

Case 1: Woo-jin

Woo-jin is a 33-year-old South Korean public policy graduate student who enrolled at a local university 9 months ago. During his first semester, he kept to himself. He received average grades in his statistical courses, but failing grades in his reading seminars, so the college assigned him a tutor for the second semester. Woo-jin has attended tutoring sessions only sporadically, and when he arrives, he is often late and poorly groomed. Although he says little, when he does speak, it is often about how his classmates are conspiring against him. To clarify what is going on, you seek the assistance of an interpreter to speak with him in his primary language. When you ask him for evidence of this conspiracy, he alludes to information he deduced from course readings and the plot of a *chang-*

geuk with which you are unfamiliar. When you seek evidence, he shows you a page from a social networking site on his phone as evidence and becomes upset as he discusses it, but all you can see are invitations to lectures and concerned messages from study partners. As Woo-jin speaks, you find it progressively harder to understand him because he shifts from one topic to another without a clear connection. When you ask about his grades, he admits they are even worse this semester but blames the government. When you ask if the situation has gotten so bad that he wants to return to his home country, he shrugs his shoulders and admits that his own government is conspiring against him as well. He shakes his head when you ask if he is depressed, but he exhibits a flat affect and often appears to be engaged in an internal conversation. He denies any history of manic or depressive episodes. You prescribe a medication to treat psychosis. When he returns 1 week later, he cannot sit still in your office, rocking from foot to foot and pacing around the room.

The essential criteria for schizophrenia and its time course remain the same in DSM-5-TR. For these criteria to be met, a person must have been experiencing continuous signs of disturbance for at least 6 months and two or more of the following symptoms for at least 1 month: delusions, hallucinations, disorganized speech, grossly abnormal psychomotor behavior, and negative symptoms. At least one of the disturbances must be one of the condition's core symptoms: delusions, hallucinations, or disorganized speech. When a patient is being interviewed, a belief that is idiosyncratic and deeply held is not necessarily delusional, and the authors of DSM-5-TR have revived attention to the difference between delusions and strongly held ideas.

Clinicians must be especially attentive to such differences, according to DSM-5-TR, whenever a patient has a different cultural, religious, or linguistic background from the interviewer. A prudent clinician will not pathologize difference qua difference. For example, a widely held religious belief from one culture can appear delusional when isolated as a symptom in a clinical encounter, especially when elicited in translation. Alternately, increased religious activity or heightened beliefs may be most consistent with a psychotic experience. Similarly, paranoia can be psychosis or a normal response to torture, violence, or discrimination.

DSM-5-TR has specific advice for the diagnostic interview, encouraging interviewers struggling to distinguish between odd and psychotic beliefs to assess if seemingly odd beliefs are grounded in reality, linked to an external stimulus, coherent and goal-directed, and communicated with an appropriate range of affective, motor, and verbal behavior. I find it helpful to perform reality testing or even formal thought records with patients to explore how they structure their days, how they name a distressing event, and how they experience and interpret an event (see, e.g., Cupitt 2019). If a belief meets all of these criteria, it is less likely to be a psychotic belief. If you are still struggling to determine whether a belief is delusional, consider using the Cultural Formulation Interview, which is discussed in Chapter 12, "Selected DSM-5-TR Assessment Measures." In this way, DSM-5-TR attends to cultural variations and helps us distinguish the normal but unfamiliar from the pathological.

DSM-5-TR also renews attention to the functional consequences of having a psychotic disorder. For example, the authors of DSM-5-TR observe that among people with schizophrenia the deficits in reading ability are more profound than other cognitive deficits, which may explain Woo-jin's differential academic performance in statistical versus seminar reading courses. An interviewer must carefully distinguish if Woo-jin's academic failure is a knowledge deficit, an artifact of learning in a second language, or the kind of acquired dyslexia that often accompanies a psychotic disorder.

A person with schizophrenia can be diagnosed with a specific time course (first vs. multiple episodes; partial vs. full remission; and an acute vs. continuous acute episode) that can also now be potentially described either as having prominent negative features or as occurring with catatonia. Catatonia can also be diagnosed dimensionally, as an experience within the context of a neurodevelopmental, bipolar, or depressive disorder, or other medical conditions. The dimensional system also allows for acknowledgment of concomitant disturbances in cognition, depression, and mania in a person diagnosed with schizophrenia using the Clinician-Rated Dimensions of Psychosis Symptom Severity, included in Chapter 12.

When a patient experiences an adverse effect of a treatment, a clinician can diagnose one of the medication-induced movement disorders and other adverse effects of medication included within DSM-5-TR. Many of these adverse effects, like the medication-induced acute akathisia experienced by Woo-jin, can be provoked by the medications commonly used to treat a person with a psychotic disorder. When a clinician carefully diagnoses these adverse effects, they engage in person-centered care, increase medication concordance, and improve future treatment.

Finally, the authors of DSM-5 also made changes to several diagnoses related to schizophrenia.

Within Section III, attenuated psychotic syndrome was rewritten to focus on its core symptoms: attenuated delusions, attenuated hallucinations, and attenuated disorganized speech. Along with its accompanying text, this diagnosis allows a clinician to recognize a person with reasonable insight whose psychotic symptoms are less severe and more transient. Woojin is the right age to experience an attenuated psychotic syndrome, but his symptoms are severe and he is unable to appreciate that his perceptions are altered, making this diagnosis less likely.

Substance/medication-induced psychotic disorder observes that a person can experience delusions or hallucinations after intoxication or withdrawal from either a substance or a medication. DSM-5-TR also includes evidence from the research literature that the psychosis induced by some substances, like cannabis, is associated with the subsequent development of a chronic psychotic disorder.

Case 2: Ruth

Ruth is a 56-year-old teacher with no past psychiatric history who reports that for 3 weeks she has been unable to sleep because she has been hearing the voice of her deceased husband asking her, "Why didn't you care for me?" She occasionally hears his baritone voice during the day as well. He died of a heart attack 2 months ago while they were attending the wedding of the youngest of their three children. Ruth had approved of the wedding, but now wonders if the relationship has been cursed by her own husband's death. Ruth and her husband had enjoyed a close relationship, and they had been looking forward to celebrating their 30th anniversary later in the year. Although her husband had high cholesterol and hypertension, Ruth was surprised by his death and worries that she "should have seen it coming. I should have saved him. I knew he needed to take better care of himself. It's like I killed him." She feels profoundly guilty about his death, especially at night, when she is unable to sleep more than a couple of hours. She says, "I feel like I am finally going mishegas." She denies thoughts of suicide but wonders frequently if her life is still worth living. She describes her mood as "down," reports poor energy, and appears fatigued. She admits that her appetite is decreased and shrugs her shoulders when asked if she has lost weight, but her clothes appear loose-fitting. She says she has been attending to her grieving family and participating in services at her synagogue, and has returned to work last week, but feels disinterested and distracted. Ruth denies any previous depressive, hypomanic, or manic episodes and drinks alcohol only at social events.

The main criteria for major depressive disorder have remained stable since DSM-IV. A depressive episode is still defined by the presence of five or more of the following symptoms during the same 2-week period: an enduringly depressed mood, anhedonia, significant weight loss or weight gain, insomnia or hypersomnia, psychomotor agitation or retardation, fatigue or loss of energy, feelings of worthlessness or excessive guilt, diminished concentration, and recurrent thoughts of death or suicide. An episode must include depressed mood or anhedonia, cause significant distress, and not be caused by substance use or another medical condition.

What is different in DSM-5-TR?

First, Ruth clearly associates her depression with the death of her husband. In DSM-5, her presentation might not meet criteria for a major depressive episode because it could be considered bereavement, which is itself a kind of culturally conditioned illness. This exclusion is removed in DSM-5-TR.

Bereavement, or grief, signals a strong attachment that is an appropriate response; people are, after all, constituted by their relationships. Within DSM-5-TR, grief is distinguished from major depressive disorder in several ways. Grieving people typically experience episodic depressive thoughts when thinking about the deceased, are preoccupied with memories of the deceased, and often preserve their own self-esteem and sense of humor. A person experiencing a major depressive episode will, by contrast, experience persistent depressive thoughts even when not thinking about the deceased, are preoccupied by self-critical thoughts, often experience worthlessness, and typically lose their sense of humor. Ruth's comment about going mishegas suggests she may still have her sense of humor (Neugeboren et al. 2013). Finally, while not apparently true for Ruth, who has no psychiatric history, depression in the context of bereavement is more common among people vulnerable to depression. Based on her symptoms, Ruth's presentation meets the criteria for major depressive disorder, single episode.

Second, the specifiers for her diagnosis are different in DSM-5-TR. An episode of depression can now be specified as being with psychotic features but as not being severe. In DSM-IV, the presence of psychotic symptoms necessarily meant the episode was severe. Because Ruth is still working and attending to her family, her episode could be classified as moderate using DSM-5-TR, but with psychotic features because she is hearing the voice of her deceased husband.

Third, Ruth's experience can be distinguished from prolonged grief disorder, a new diagnosis within DSM-5-TR. If a person is persistently grieving—at least 12 months for adults and 6 months for a child or adolescent—after the death of someone they were close to, a clinician should consider this new diagnosis. The death of Ruth's husband is too recent for this diagnosis. In addition, the symptoms of prolonged grief disorder do not match Ruth's experience. A persistently grieving person experiences, nearly daily, intense yearning or longing for the deceased or preoccupation with thoughts or memories of the deceased that exceeds expected cultural or social norms. This diagnosis also requires that one experience three or more of the following symptoms nearly daily for the last month: identity disruption; marked sense of disbelief about the death; avoidance of reminders that the person is dead; intense emotional pain; difficulty reintegrating into activities and relationships; emotional numbness; feeling that life is meaningless; intense loneliness.

DSM-5-TR provides several ways to characterize the experience of a person who, like Ruth, has experienced a change in mood after the loss of a beloved person.

Case 3: Roberto

Roberto is a 47-year-old man who volunteers for a research trial exploring novel treatments for treatment-refractory depression. When you screen Roberto during an initial telepsychiatry encounter, he seems distant. He volunteers little about himself but on direct questioning reports feeling "down" a couple of times each week, usually "after some bad event at work." No one has ever told him that he seemed agitated. He denies significant weight loss. He reports that it takes him a "little longer" to get to sleep but denies frank insomnia. He reports that he has "less energy than I used to" but when pressed admits that it mostly takes him longer to complete tasks that he used to perform quickly. He describes decreased decisiveness. He denies suicidal ideation. He reports that he has lost interest in his work, which he used to enjoy, but attributes it chiefly to "increased conflict with my boss over late work assignments." Roberto denies a history of manic or psychotic symptoms. He was previously treated for depression 20 years ago but denies any subsequent episodes. Roberto drinks an "occasional" glass of wine but denies any history of alcohol or substance misuse. Reviewing the study criteria, you inform Roberto that he is not a candidate for your research trial and suggest he see a local psychiatrist.

At their first meeting, Roberto reports that he was diagnosed with HIV 20 years ago but "went on and off the treatment because I hate taking pills." He denies other medical history and has never had surgery. Roberto graduated from a local university with above-average grades and later completed an online master's degree in business without difficulty. For the past 15 years, Roberto has worked as an accountant for a local firm. He has been promoted several times and manages several other accountants. For the past 5 years, he admits that "I have been turning to them to do more and more of the work, because I cannot seem to manage it like I used to." He scores a 21 of 30 on the MoCA (Montreal Cognitive Assessment), with the most difficulties in memory and visuospatial functioning. He is alert and fully oriented. Roberto lives with his long-time partner, Marc. They share the cooking, but Roberto manages their bills while his partner keeps their house. Roberto's serum B_{12}, folate, CBC, chem 7, and TSH are all within normal limits. His CD4 count is 150.

The development of a neurocognitive disorder is an object lesson in the importance of dimensional diagnostic models. By their nature, neurocognitive disorders exist along a spectrum of cognitive impairment, from a person's adult peak to their descent into dependence.

DSM-5-TR allows a clinician to observe cognitive changes in many ways. A cognitive change can be a normal component of aging and diagnosed using the ICD Z code for age-related cognitive decline. A cognitive change can also occur within the context of another mental disorder, like schizophrenia, major depressive disorder, or a substance use disorder.

A cognitive change can also be discrete or global. DSM-5-TR includes a clinically essential table that lists cognitive domains, provides examples of symptoms, and describes the assessments a clinician can use. So, for example, with a patient like Roberto, who is experiencing deficits in learning and memory, DSM-5-TR suggests ways to assess both his immediate memory span (repeating a list of words or digits) and recent memory (either through free recall, cued recall, or recognition memory). Assessing a particular cognitive domain is essential for determining which neurocognitive disorder is being experienced by a patient.

The core neurocognitive disorders are delirium and major and mild neurocognitive disorder.

Delirium is a disturbance in attention accompanied by a reduced awareness of the environment. Additional cognitive disturbances—in language, memory, orientation, perception, and visuospatial ability—are also experienced. Delirium typically develops over a period of hours to a few days and is a direct physiological consequence of a medical condition, substance use, or toxin exposure. Since treating the underlying physiological cause is essential to treatment, DSM-5-TR provides specifiers to name the course and associated behavior, as it does with most disorders, but also the causative agent.

This is a signal advance for a diagnostic system based on symptoms. When we know the etiology of a mental disorder, the authors of DSM-5-TR ask clinicians to identify the cause.

As a result, the diagnosis of mild and major neurocognitive disorder often follows a three-step process.

First, a clinician should carefully assess a patient for the presence of cognitive decline that interferes with everyday activities. The diagnosis requires a significant cognitive decline in one or more cognitive domains and a substantial impairment in cognitive performance. The diagnosis should not be made if the cognitive decline occurs only in the context of delirium or another mental disorder. To make the diagnosis, the clinician should ideally include information from people who know a patient well; in the case of Roberto, you need to speak with Marc. It is also ideal to perform a validated clinical assessment of cognition.

Second, a clinician needs to assess how profoundly the decline interferes with everyday activities. When a person's cognitive decline does not compromise their independence, a clinician should diagnose a mild neurocognitive disorder. A patient with this degree of impairment may need increased effort, compensatory strategies, or accommodations to accomplish daily tasks. By contrast, when a person's cognitive decline compromises their independence, a clinician should diagnose a major neurocognitive disorder. When you speak with Marc, you want to ask about how well Roberto does on more complex activities like paying bills and taking medications.

Third, a clinician should identify the cause of a patient's neurocognitive disorder. The authors of DSM-5-TR ask clinicians to specify if a patient's neurocognitive disorder is due to Alzheimer's, frontotemporal degeneration, Lewy body disease, vascular disease, traumatic brain injury, substance/medication use, HIV infection, prion disease, or Parkinson's disease. Using these specifiers drives clinical action because in addition to different symptoms and courses, these conditions have different treatments. In the case of Roberto, whose neurocognitive disorder is most likely caused by an HIV infection, a proper diagnosis would encourage a clinician to prescribe effective antiretroviral therapy and to screen for associated conditions, both of which are discussed in the text of DSM-5-TR.

The cognitive domain, degree of functional impairment, and the cause of each neurocognitive disorder vary. DSM-5-TR encourages you to identify each so that you can effect change for a person like Roberto.

Case 4: Keith

Keith is a 33-year-old assistant professor who has just been denied tenure despite having written what he calls "the best dissertation in my field in the last century." After receiving notice that he would not receive tenure, Keith angrily quit his position. He has sought legal counsel to sue his former university, but says, "None of the attorneys I have contacted is sufficiently well trained to represent me," insisting that they would need a doctorate in his own field as well as a legal degree "from a top-five research university" to grasp his situation. You are meeting with Keith because an attorney suggested you might assist him in crafting an appropriate strategy. Keith begins the meeting by asking about your training and asking for copies "of your 10 most important papers." He denies manic, depressive, and psychotic symptoms, and insists that his only problem is that "other people cannot understand me." He was previously engaged to marry but broke it off because "she was not distinguished enough." His current girlfriend, he tells you, has "strong breeding," but he admits that he frequently yells at her when they are out in public when he feels she does not give him the proper attention. According to Keith they fight less in private, because "I am a chivalrous man: meek at the table, stern at the battle." When asked about alcohol and substance use, he says, "I am above drugs but can hold my drink." He reports craving for, and tolerance to, alcohol. When asked if he has close friends, he names several historical figures, saying, "Those are the kind of people whom I see as my peers." When asked about his colleagues at the university, he complains that they were too "envious of me to be true peers."

In DSM-5-TR, personality disorders can be diagnosed by one of two systems. The first system is a categorical system familiar to any experienced interviewer. This system is in the main text of DSM-5-TR and is endorsed for regular clinical use; it is also the system used in Chapters 3 and 6 of this guide. The second system is a dimensional system. This system is the "Emerging Measures and Models" of DSM-5-TR and is endorsed for research use. We can consider Keith's presentation using both systems.

In the categorical model endorsed for clinical work, Keith's presentation clearly meets the criteria for narcissistic personality disorder. He endorses at least five of the enumerated manifestations of this personality disorder. DSM-5-TR renews our attention to the vulnerability that a person like Keith often experiences—internal self-doubt, self-criticism, and emptiness—and the association with various levels of functional impairment and with suicidal ideation when a person with this personality structure is exposed to imperfection and failure.

DSM-5-TR still lists 10 specific personality disorders, and the symptomatic manifestations of each disorder remain unchanged. The general definition of a personality disorder remains "an enduring pattern of inner experience and behavior that deviates markedly from the norms and expectations of the individual's culture" (American Psychiatric Association 2022, p. 733). The personality disorders are organized into Cluster A, for people who often appear odd or eccentric; Cluster B, for people who often appear dramatic, emotional, or erratic; and Cluster C, for people who often appear anxious or fearful.

In short, DSM-5-TR endorses a diagnostic system for clinical use in which personality disorders are organized based on appearances. The authors acknowledge that even when used properly, their current categorical system often leads to the diagnosis of multiple personality disorders in the same person and use of the other specified and unspecified personality disorder diagnoses.

To address these problems, DSM-5-TR characterizes a dimensional approach, based on underlying psychological traits, as a future way to identify personality disorders.

The dimensional approach is a remarkable change in the categorical features and conceptualization of personality disorders. On a practical level, the DSM-5-TR personality disorder work group removed four personality disorders—paranoid, schizoid, histrionic, and dependent—after determining that they lacked sufficient evidence for their utility and validity. The DSM-5-TR work group found enough evidence to support the retention of only six categorical DSM-5-TR personality disorders—antisocial, avoidant, borderline, narcissistic, obsessive-compulsive, and schizotypal—and refined their diagnostic criteria thoroughly. In general, the work group reduced attention to behavior in the categorical diagnoses of personality disorders in favor of assessing functional impairments. In short, they encourage diagnosing a personality disorder only when a person has an impaired ability to establish a coherent identity, to be self-directed, to develop empathy for others, and to develop reciprocal relationships. You still identify pathological personality traits, but only after first establishing whether the patient has impairment in self-functioning and interpersonal functioning.

The authors of DSM-5-TR designed this dimensional approach to limit the diagnosis of personality disorders to those with the strongest evidence base, to reduce the diagnosis of multiple personality disorders in a single person, and to remove the diagnosis of personality disorder not otherwise specified. With the dimensional model, you can diagnose one of the six personality disorders named above and specify additional traits for each, or you can use a new diagnosis, personality disorder—trait specified (e.g., personality disorder—antagonism, which is described below), to indicate the presence of specific traits that do not reach the level of a particular diagnosis.

Keith's example illustrates several of these changes. In the categorical model retained in DSM-5-TR, an arbitrary number of personality traits lead to a diagnosis. In DSM-5-TR's proposed dimensional model, the diagnosis of narcissistic personality disorder begins with impairments in self-functioning and interpersonal functioning. For the criteria to be met, Keith must have impairment in self-functioning as indicated either by excessive reference to others for self-definition and self-esteem or by goal setting based on gaining approval from others. He must also have impairment in interpersonal functioning as indicated by a lack of empathy or an inability to experience emotionally intimate relationships with others. Unlike in earlier models of personality disorders, these functional impairments are common to all personality disorders. If a patient endorses these impairments in self-functioning and interpersonal functioning, the interviewer is prompted to characterize which pathological personality traits are present. I model this in Chapter 13, "Dimensional Diagnosis of Personality Disorders." If we use this model to consider Keith's presentation, the pathological personality traits are grandiosity and attention-seeking.

Grandiosity and attention-seeking are what the DSM-5-TR dimensional model calls "facets" of antagonism, one of the Five Factors used as an organizing principle for personality disorder diagnoses. In the literature, *Five-Factor Model* usually refers to the five strength-based adaptive personality traits of *neuroticism, extraversion, agreeableness, conscientiousness,* and *openness to experience* (Digman 1990). Because the DSM-5 work group built their diagnostic criteria from a deficit-based, rather than strength-based, model, they organized personality disorders around five companion maladaptive traits: *negative affectivity, detachment, antagonism, disinhibition,* and *psychoticism.* The authors found compelling evidence for these five maladaptive traits as stable and predictive of problems in self-functioning and interpersonal functioning. In addition, they identified "facets" for each of these five maladaptive traits. In total, DSM-5-TR enumerates 25 facets organized into five domains for each of the maladaptive traits listed above. The Five-Factor Model provides an alternative to the cluster model of categorical personality disorders, in which the latter are organized into Cluster A, B, and C disorders.

The presence of *grandiosity* and *attention-seeking* is necessary but not sufficient for a diagnosis of narcissistic personality disorder in the dimensional model. To make the diagnosis, you need to find evidence of impairment in self-functioning and interpersonal functioning. The authors of DSM-5-TR provide a 5-point scale, ranging from 0 (little or no impairment) to 4 (extreme impairment), that they call the *Level of Personality Functioning Scale,* which is included in Chapter 13 of this guidebook. This scale is an example of a dimensional assessment directly incorporated into diagnostic criteria in an effort to diagnose patients only when the diagnosis has the greatest predictive power of dysfunction. Based on their analysis of the data, the DSM-5-TR authors conclude that the presence of personality traits is most meaningful when a patient is experiencing profound impairment in self-functioning and interpersonal functioning. In the instance of Keith, even this brief sketch of his life suggests that his narcissistic traits are interfering, at the very least, with his work and romantic life. After a thorough assessment, his level of impairment would likely be scored as a 4 (Extreme Impairment) on the Level of Personality Functioning Scale.

However, if Keith had presented with self-functioning and interpersonal functioning impairments sufficient to meet criteria for a personality disorder but had not exhibited the specific traits associated with a named personality disorder, he would have been diagnosed with a personality disorder—trait specified in the dimensional model. Using the five domains named above, you could conduct a personality overview sufficient to specify a trait and make the diagnosis. If doing so would guide your diagnosis and treatment, you could alternatively use the 25 trait facets to create a personality profile in addition to the diagnosis. This process, using the Personality Trait Rating Form, is described in Chapter 13.

In reading about it, this process might seem confusing. Its merit is that it limits named personality disorders to those with the greatest validity and utility, requires evidence of serious impairment in self-functioning and interpersonal functioning, and implicitly defines healthy personality functioning, all while allowing you to make a diagnosis when evaluating someone with such impairments even if all the criteria for a specific diagnosis are not met. The authors of DSM-5-TR conceive of the dimensional diagnosis of a personality disorder as occurring in a stepwise process, beginning with determining whether a patient's presentation meets criteria for a personality disorder. This determination is based on 1) the extent to which they experience impairments in self-functioning and interpersonal functioning and 2) the extent to which their presentation meets criteria for one of the six named personality disorders or, finally, for personality disorder—trait specified, listing whichever of the five maladaptive traits (negative affectivity, detachment, antagonism, disinhibition, and psychoticism) the patient expresses. These changes in the diagnostic process for personality disorders are an attempt to use the best evidence available, while being flexible enough for clinical practice, and are reflected in the operationalized criteria presented in Chapter 13 of this guide.

Finally, the authors of DSM-5-TR recognize that a person's mental well-being is affected by environmental, material, and social conditions, which a clinician may need to address in order to improve a patient's mental health. Several of these are represented with the ICD Z codes found in DSM-5-TR's "Other Conditions That May Be a Focus of Clinical Attention" and at the end of Chapter 6 of this guide. For Keith, a clinician might consider "Spouse or Partner Abuse, Psychological" as a way to recognize that Keith's treatment of his girlfriend should be addressed in treatment. When we diagnose well, we can help a person like Keith get the actual approval and admiration they need, while improving their relations with others (see, e.g., Gabbard and Crisp 2018).

Reordered Disorders

The authors of DSM-5-TR also integrate developmental and temperamental considerations into the organization of the manual.

In previous DSM versions, disorders were grouped by their usual age at onset: during infancy, childhood, adolescence, or adulthood. The authors of DSM-5-TR instead organized disorders by common phenomenology and pathology rather than by age at onset. As a result, disorders that are most often diagnosed in children, such as separation anxiety disorder or pica, are found alongside their respective pathological neighbors—in these cases, anxiety disorders and feeding and eating disorders, respectively—but occur earlier in the chapter, just as they present earlier in life. In addition, the DSM-5-TR criteria for a condition most commonly diagnosed in adults, such as an anxiety disorder or depressive disorder, include additional information about how development influences the onset, presentation, and course of the disorder. The goal is to show how a person might experience a mental disorder differently during various developmental stages. To further emphasize a developmental perspective, the authors of DSM-5-TR present pathological categories in roughly the order in which they present, beginning with neurodevelopmental disorders and ending with paraphilic disorders.

The authors of DSM-5-TR also group the disorder categories by the presence of either internalizing or externalizing factors. Disorders associated with internalizing factors, such as depressive disorders and anxiety disorders, are presented earlier in DSM-5-TR. They are followed by disorders associated with externalizing factors, such as antisocial and elimination disorders, because the authors implicitly point to future editions in which psychiatric disorders will likely be organized by their underlying dysfunction. In a similar way, DSM-5-TR includes the etiology for several neurocognitive disorders. As the causes of mental disorders are identified, future versions of DSM will similarly identify them in the diagnostic criteria.

Finally, "unspecified" and "other specified" criteria are found in each chapter of DSM-5-TR. In general, interviewers are advised to consider "unspecified" diagnoses when a person experiences symptoms characteristic of a mental disorder that cause clinically significant distress but do not meet full criteria for a named diagnosis. If an interviewer wishes to communicate the specific reason a person does not meet criteria, the interviewer is encouraged to use the "other specified" diagnosis. For example, a person who experiences persistent auditory hallucinations in the absence of other features of schizophrenia would be diagnosed with other specified schizophrenia spectrum and other psychotic disorder (persistent auditory hallucinations). DSM-5-TR adds the diagnosis of "Unspecified Mood Disorder" for when a clinician cannot distinguish between unspecified bipolar and depressive disorders, as may occur when a patient is acutely agitated.

Conclusion

The authors of DSM-5-TR revised the text accompanying every diagnosis and, when necessary, corresponding diagnostic criteria to reflect recent advances. In this chapter, I demonstrated how the criteria and the conceptualization have changed for each of four sample diagnoses, selected for discussion because of their importance in clinical practice. Considering these four representative diagnoses illustrates the difficult task faced by the authors of DSM-5-TR in using the best available data while creating useful diagnostic criteria.

Our diagnoses must have utility so they can be formulas for clinical action.

In making diagnoses, we shape patients and practitioners alike. If, at various points in the last two centuries, our diagnostic systems were designed alternately for the asylum, battlefield, outpatient clinic, or research university (e.g., Grob 1991; Houts 2000), the diagnostic system of the future will likely be designed for the mental health practitioner who works as a consultant, diagnosing efficiently so they may initiate treatment. In the following chapter, I offer one way to do so.

Chapter 6

The DSM-5-TR
Diagnostic Interview

In Chapter 3, "The 30-Minute Diagnostic Interview," I outlined a diagnostic interview that included a screening question for each of the DSM-5-TR categories of mental disorders. If a person answers affirmatively to one of those questions, what do you do? In this chapter, I demonstrate how the screening questions are the avenues of the psychiatric diagnostic interview. A good interviewer skillfully travels these avenues with a patient and, when possible, reaches a specific and accurate diagnosis along the way.

This chapter follows the order of DSM-5-TR disorders, beginning with neurodevelopmental disorders. For each category of DSM-5-TR diagnoses presented, whether bipolar disorders or elimination disorders, the section begins with one or more screening questions from the model interview presented in Chapter 3. After the screening questions, there are follow-up questions. If the follow-up questions include a measure of impairment or a measure of time, these measures are a required part of the subsequent diagnostic criteria. By putting follow-up questions before the additional symptom questions in the diagnostic criteria, I am attempting to make the interview more efficient and precise while reserving full diagnosis of a mental disorder for a person who is impaired by their experiences.

The screening and follow-up questions are followed by the diagnostic criteria. When the diagnostic criteria are to be elicited by the interviewer, I offer italicized prompts for the relevant symptom. I structured these questions so that an affirmative answer meets the criteria for that symptom. When the diagnostic criteria are observed rather than elicited, as in the case of disorganized speech or psychomotor retardation or autonomic hyperactivity, they are listed as instructions to the interviewer, set in roman type. The minimum number of symptoms necessary to reach a particular diagnosis is underlined. Questions specifically included for children and adolescents are shaded. Of course, I do not list all the possible questions that can be used to elicit a relevant symptom, but these questions are specifically designed to follow DSM-5-TR. To make the diagnostic process as clear as possible, I have included negative criteria for a DSM-5-TR diagnosis under the heading "Exclusion." For example, DSM-5-TR observes that a person's presentation does not meet criteria for schizophrenia if they experience psychotic symptoms only as the physiological effect of a substance. These exclusion criteria usually do not require you to ask a specific question, but instead depend on the history you elicit. The most common subtypes, specifiers, and severity measures are listed under the heading "Modifiers."

In the interest of brevity, this guide includes diagnostic questions for the most common DSM-5-TR disorders. The idea is to focus on learning the diagnostic criteria for the paradigmatic disorders in each section before exploring the related diagnoses—that is, to know the main streets of DSM-5-TR before learning its side streets.

In this book, the side streets are labeled as "alternatives," a term that is not used in DSM-5-TR. These alternatives include only related diagnoses from the same DSM-5-TR chapter. For example, adjustment disorder is listed as an alternative to posttraumatic stress disorder (PTSD), because they are grouped together in DSM-5-TR. In contrast, traumatic brain injury and other diagnoses listed in the differential diagnosis for PTSD are not in the "alternatives" section for PTSD, because they are found in different sections of DSM-5-TR. For each diagnosis listed in "alternatives," the essential diagnostic criteria are included and the interviewer is referred to the corresponding pages in DSM-5-TR to read the diagnostic criteria and associated material in detail.

Although this guide includes all the diagnoses within DSM-5-TR, it eliminates repetitive criteria, especially for the various mental disorders associated with another medical condition or substance-induced mental disorders, in which, broadly, the symptoms of a disorder are present as a direct effect of another medical condition or a substance.

As this overview suggests, this book is no substitute for DSM-5-TR, but it serves as a practical diagnostic tool, an operationalized version of DSM-5-TR—the equivalent of the sketched version of a city street that a phone's map displays, rather than the detailed portrait of each side street. This book will help you reach your destination in a timely fashion but without the rich detail of DSM-5-TR. In the abstract, this diagnostic interview process may sound confusing; however, once you start with a common diagnosis (say, bipolar disorder) and practice the process a few times, the organization will be clear.

Neurodevelopmental Disorders

DSM-5-TR pp. 35–99

Screening questions for a person (or caregiver): *Did you have any behavioral or learning problems during your early childhood? When you started school, did you have trouble relating socially or keeping up academically with your classmates because of behavioral or learning problems?*

   If yes, ask: *Do you have trouble concentrating or struggle with being impulsive or hyperactive? Do you have difficulty communicating with other people or in social interactions? Are there specific bothersome behaviors that you do frequently and find hard to control? Do you struggle to learn, more than your classmates do?*

- If deficits in intellectual functioning or specific academic skills predominate, proceed to intellectual developmental disorder (intellectual disability) criteria.
- If deficits in social interactions or impairing motor behaviors predominate, proceed to autism spectrum disorder criteria.
- If inattention, hyperactivity, or impulsivity predominate, proceed to attention-deficit/hyperactivity disorder criteria.

1. Intellectual Developmental Disorder (Intellectual Disability)

   a. Inclusion: Requires intellectual deficits, beginning during the developmental period, that impair adaptive function as manifested by <u>both</u> of the following symptoms.

      i. Deficits in intellectual functions, such as reasoning, problem solving, planning, abstract thinking, judgment, academic learning, and experiential learning. Must be confirmed by both clinical assessment and individualized, standardized intelligence testing.
      ii. Impaired adaptive functioning, normalized for developmental and sociocultural standards, which

restricts participation and performance in one or more aspects of daily life activities. The limitations result in the need for ongoing support at school, at work, or for independent life.

b. Modifiers

    i. Severity (see DSM-5-TR, pp. 39–41, Table 1)

- Mild
- Moderate
- Severe
- Profound

c. Alternatives

    i. If a person younger than 5 years fails to meet expected developmental milestones in several areas of intellectual functioning and is unable to undergo systematic assessments of intellectual functioning, consider global developmental delay (see DSM-5-TR, p. 46). This diagnosis requires eventual reassessment.

    ii. If a person older than 5 years exhibits intellectual disability that cannot be well characterized because of associated sensory or physical impairments, consider unspecified intellectual developmental disorder (see DSM-5-TR, p. 46). This diagnosis should be used only in exceptional circumstances and requires eventual reassessment.

    iii. If a person has persistent difficulties in the acquisition and use of language (spoken, written, sign, or other modalities) that begin in the early developmental period and result in substantial functional limitations, consider the diagnosis of language disorder (full criteria are available in DSM-5-TR, p. 47). Language disorder occurs as a primary impairment or may coexist with other disorders. This diagnosis should not be used if the language difficulties are better explained by hearing or sensory impairment, intellectual developmental disorder, or global developmental delay or are caused by another medical or neurological condition.

    iv. If a person has persistent difficulties in speech sound production that interfere with speech intelligibility or prevent verbal communication of messages, consider speech sound disorder (full criteria are available in

DSM-5-TR, p. 50). The symptoms must be present in the early developmental period and result in limitations in effective communication, social participation, academic achievement, and occupational performance, individually or in any combination. Speech sound disorder occurs as a primary impairment or coexists with other disorders or congenital or acquired conditions. This diagnosis should not be used if the speech sound difficulties are due to congenital or acquired medical or neurological conditions.

v. If a person has marked and frequent disturbances in the fluency and time patterning of speech that are inappropriate for the person's age and language skills, consider childhood-onset fluency disorder (stuttering) (full criteria are available in DSM-5-TR, pp. 51–52). Symptoms must begin in the early developmental period. The disturbance must cause anxiety about speaking or the ability to communicate effectively. This disorder can coexist with other disorders. However, the diagnosis should not be used if the disorder is attributable to a speech-motor or sensory deficit, is attributable to another medical or neurological condition, or is better explained by another mental disorder.

vi. If a person has persistent difficulties in the social use of verbal and nonverbal communication that functionally limit effective communication, social participation, social relationships, academic achievement, or occupational performance, consider social (pragmatic) communication disorder (full criteria are available in DSM-5-TR, p. 54). Symptoms begin during the early developmental period. The disorder can coexist with other disorders. However, this diagnosis should not be used if the symptoms are better explained by intellectual developmental disorder, global developmental delay, or another mental disorder or are attributable to another medical or neurological condition.

vii. If a person has symptoms of a communication disorder that cause clinically significant distress or impairment but do not meet the full criteria for a communication disorder or another neurodevelopmental disorder, consider unspecified communication disorder (see DSM-5-TR, p. 56).

viii. If a person has persistent difficulties in learning and using academic skills that begin during school-age years and eventually result in significant interference with academic or occupational performance, consider specific learning disorder (full criteria, along with severity ratings, are available in DSM-5-TR, pp. 76–78). To meet criteria, the current skills must be well below the average range for the person's age, gender, cultural group, and level of education. The symptoms must not be better accounted for by another intellectual, medical, mental, neurological, or sensory disorder.

2. Autism Spectrum Disorder

   a. Inclusion: Requires persistent deficits in social communication and social interaction, across multiple contexts, that are present in the early developmental period but that may not be manifest until social demands exceed limited capacities, and that cause clinically significant impairment in functioning. The disorder is marked by, for example, <u>all</u> of the following persistent deficits in social communication and interaction.

       i. Deficits in social-emotional reciprocity: *When you meet someone, how do you introduce yourself? Do you find it hard to greet another person? Do you find it hard to share your interests, thoughts, and feelings with other people? Do you dislike to hear about what other people are interested in or how they feel?*

       ii. Deficits in nonverbal communicative behaviors used for social interaction; these are usually observed by the interviewer and range from poorly integrated verbal and nonverbal communication, through abnormalities in eye contact and body language, or deficits in understanding and use of nonverbal communication, to total lack of facial expression or gestures.

       iii. Deficits in developing and maintaining relationships: *Are you disinterested in other people? Are you unable to engage in imaginative play with other people? Do you find it difficult to make new friends? When the situation around you changes, do you find it hard to adjust your own behavior in response?*

b. Inclusion: In addition, the diagnosis requires at least <u>two</u> of the following signs of restricted, repetitive patterns of behavior, interests, or activities.

    i. Stereotyped or repetitive speech, motor movements, or use of objects, such as simple motor stereotypies, echolalia, repetitive use of objects, or idiosyncratic phrases.

    ii. Insistence on sameness and excessive adherence to routines or avoidance of change: *Do you have any special routines or patterns of behavior? What happens when you cannot follow these routines or engage in these behaviors? Do you struggle to change?*

    iii. Restricted interests of abnormal intensity or focus: *Do you intensely focus upon, or find yourself very interested in, just a few things?*

    iv. Hyper- or hyporeactivity to sensory input: *How do you experience something that is painful? Something hot? Something cold? Are there particular sounds, textures, or smells to which you respond strongly? Do you find yourself fascinated with lights or spinning objects?*

c. Modifiers

    i. Specifiers

- With (or without) accompanying intellectual impairment
- With (or without) accompanying language impairment
- Associated with a known genetic or other medical condition or environmental factor
- Associated with a neurodevelopmental, mental, or behavioral problem
- With catatonia

    ii. Severity is coded separately for the social communication impairments and for the restricted, repetitive patterns of behavior.

- Level 1: Requiring support
- Level 2: Requiring substantial support
- Level 3: Requiring very substantial support

d. Alternatives

    i. If a person exhibits coordinated motor performance substantially below expected levels, which significantly interferes with activities of daily living or academic achievement and which began in the early developmental period, consider developmental coordination disorder (full criteria are in DSM-5-TR, pp. 85–86). Examples include clumsiness, as well as slow and inaccurate performance of motor skills. The disturbance cannot be attributable to another medical or neurological condition or be better explained by another mental disorder.

ii. If a person exhibits repetitive, seemingly driven, yet apparently purposeless motor behavior, such as hand shaking or waving, body rocking, head banging, or self-biting, consider stereotypic movement disorder (full criteria are in DSM-5-TR, p. 89). The motor disturbance causes clinically significant distress or impairment. The motor behavior is not attributable to the physiological effects of another medical condition or a substance and is not better explained by the symptoms of another mental disorder.

iii. A tic is a sudden, rapid, recurrent, nonrhythmic motor movement or vocalization. If a person experiences both motor and vocal tics beginning before age 18 years, consider Tourette's disorder (full criteria are in DSM-5-TR, p. 93). The tics may wax and wane in frequency but must persist for at least 1 year after onset. The tics cannot be attributable to the physiological effects of another medical condition or a substance.

iv. If a person experiences either motor or vocal tics, but not both, during his illness, and has never met criteria for Tourette's disorder, consider persistent (chronic) motor or vocal tic disorder (full criteria are in DSM-5-TR, p. 93). The onset is before age 18 years, and the tics may wax and wane in frequency but must have persisted for more than 1 year since their onset.

v. If a person experiences motor and/or vocal tics for at least 1 year, beginning before age 18 years, and the tics are not attributable to the physiological consequences of another medical condition or a substance, and the criteria for Tourette's disorder or persistent (chronic) motor or vocal tic disorder have never been met, consider provisional tic disorder (full criteria are in DSM-5-TR, p. 93).

vi. If a person experiences tics that do not meet criteria for a specific tic disorder because the movements or vocalizations are atypical in relation to age at onset or clinical presentation, consider other specified or unspecified tic disorder (see DSM-5-TR, p. 98).

3. Attention-Deficit/Hyperactivity Disorder

a. Inclusion: Requires a pattern of behavior, with onset before age 12 years, that is present in multiple settings and gives rise to social, educational, or work performance difficulties. The symptoms must be persistently present for at least 6 months to a degree inconsistent with developmental level. The disorder is manifested by at least <u>six</u> of the following symptoms of inattention.

i. Overlooks details: *Over at least the last 6 months, have other people told you that you often overlook or miss details, or that you made careless mistakes in your work?*

ii. Task inattention: *Do you often have difficulty staying focused on a task or activity, such as reading a lengthy writing or listening to a lecture or conversation?*

iii. Appears not to listen: *Do other people tell you that when they speak to you, your mind often seems to be elsewhere or that it seems like you are not listening?*

iv. Fails to finish tasks: *Do you often struggle to finish schoolwork, chores, or work assignments because you lose focus or are easily sidetracked?*

v. Difficulty organizing tasks: *Do you often find it difficult to organize tasks or activities? Do you struggle with time management or fail to meet deadlines?*

vi. Avoids tasks requiring sustained mental activity: *Do you often avoid tasks that require sustained mental effort?*

vii. Often loses things necessary for tasks: *Do you often lose things that are essential for tasks or activities, such as school materials, books, tools, wallets, keys, paperwork, eyeglasses, or your phone?*

viii. Easily distracted: *Do you find that you are often easily distracted by things or thoughts unrelated to the activity or task you are supposed to be doing?*

ix. Often forgetful: *Do you find, or do other people find, that you are often forgetful in your daily activities?*

b. Inclusion: Alternatively, requires the presence of at least <u>six</u> of the following manifestations of hyperactivity and impulsivity over the same course.

i. Fidgets: *Over the last 6 months, have you often found yourself fidgeting with your hands or feet? Do you find it hard to sit without squirming?*

ii. Leaves seat: *When you are in a situation where you are expected to sit, do you often leave your seat?*

iii. Runs or climbs: *Do you often find yourself running around or climbing in a situation where doing so is inappropriate?*

iv. Unable to maintain quiet: *Do you often find yourself unable to play or engage in leisure activities quietly?*

v. Hyperactivity: *Do you often feel as if you are, or do other people describe you as always being, on the go or acting as if you were "driven by a motor"? Do you find it uncomfortable to sit still for an extended time?*

vi. Talks excessively: *Do you often talk excessively?*

vii. Blurts answers: *Do you often struggle to wait your turn in a conversation? Do you often complete other people's sentences or blurt out an answer before a question has been completed?*

viii. Struggles to take turns: *Do you often have difficulty waiting your turn or waiting in line?*

ix. Interrupts or intrudes: *Do you often butt into other people's activities, conversations, or games? Do you often start using other people's things without permission?*

c. Exclusion: If the criteria are not met in two or more settings, or there is no evidence that the symptoms interfere with functioning, the symptoms occur only in the context of a psychotic disorder, or the symptoms are better explained by another mental disorder, do not make the diagnosis.

d. Modifiers

   i. Specifiers

      • Combined presentation: If both inattention and hyperactivity-impulsivity criteria are met for the past 6 months

      • Predominantly inattentive presentation: If inattention criteria are met but hyperactivity-impulsivity criteria have not been met for the past 6 months

      • Predominantly hyperactive/impulsive presentation: If hyperactivity-impulsivity criteria are met and inattention criteria have not been met for the past 6 months

   ii. Specifiers

      • In partial remission

iii. Severity

- Mild: Few, if any, symptoms in excess of those required to make the diagnosis are present, and symptoms result in no more than minor impairments in social or occupational functioning.
- Moderate: Symptoms or functional impairment between "mild" and "severe" is present.
- Severe: Many symptoms in excess of those required to make the diagnosis, or several symptoms that are particularly severe, are present, or the symptoms result in marked impairment in social or occupational functioning.

e. Alternatives: If a person is experiencing subthreshold symptoms or you have not yet had sufficient opportunity to verify all criteria, consider other specified or unspecified attention-deficit/hyperactivity disorder (see DSM-5-TR, p. 76). The symptoms must be associated with impairment and do not occur exclusively during the course of schizophrenia or another psychotic disorder and are not better explained by another mental disorder.

Schizophrenia Spectrum and Other Psychotic Disorders

DSM-5-TR pp. 101–138

Screening questions: *Have you seen visions or other things that other people did not see? Have you heard noises, sounds, or voices that other people did not hear? Do you ever feel like people are following you or trying to hurt you in some way? Have you ever felt that you had special powers, such as reading other people's minds? While watching television or listening to music, have you ever felt that it was referring to you?*

If yes, ask: *Do these experiences influence your behavior or tell you to do things? Did these experiences ever cause you significant trouble with your friends or family, at work, or in another setting?*

- If yes, proceed to schizophrenia criteria.

1. Schizophrenia

a. Inclusion: Requires at least 6 months of continuous signs of disturbance, which may include prodromal or residual symptoms. During at least 1 month of that period, at least <u>two</u> of the following symptoms are present, and at least <u>one</u> of the symptoms must be delusions, hallucinations, or disorganized speech.

    i. Delusions: *Is anyone working to harm or hurt you? When you read a book, watch television, or use a computer, do you ever find that there are messages intended just for you? Do you have special powers or abilities?*

    ii. Hallucinations: *When you are awake, do you ever hear a voice different from your own thoughts that other people cannot hear? When you are awake, do you ever see things that other people cannot see?*

    iii. Disorganized speech like frequent derailment or incoherence

    iv. Grossly disorganized or catatonic behavior

    v. Negative symptoms such as diminished emotional expression or avolition

b. Exclusion: If the disturbance is attributable to the physiological effects of a substance (e.g., a drug of abuse, a medication) or another medical condition, do not make the diagnosis.

c. Exclusion: If a person has been diagnosed with autism spectrum disorder or a communication disorder of childhood onset, schizophrenia may be diagnosed only if prominent delusions or hallucinations are also present for at least 1 month.

d. Modifiers

    i. Specifiers

- First episode, currently in acute episode
- First episode, currently in partial remission
- First episode, currently in full remission
- Multiple episodes, currently in acute episode
- Multiple episodes, currently in partial remission
- Multiple episodes, currently in full remission
- Continuous
- Unspecified

    ii. Additional specifier

- With catatonia: Use when at least <u>three</u> of the following are present: stupor, catalepsy, waxy flexibility, mutism, negativism, posturing, mannerisms, stereotypies, agitation, grimacing, echolalia, echopraxia.

iii. Severity

  • Severity is rated by a quantitative assessment of the primary symptoms of psychosis, each of which may be rated for its current severity on a five-point scale (see Chapter 12, "Selected DSM-5-TR Assessment Measures," pp. 225–230).

e. Alternatives

  i. If a person has a pervasive pattern of eccentric behaviors, cognitive and perceptual distortions, and little capacity for close relationships, consider schizotypal personality disorder (full criteria are in DSM-5-TR, pp. 744–745). If the disturbance occurs exclusively in the context of schizophrenia, a depressive or manic episode with psychotic features, or autism spectrum disorder, do not make the diagnosis.

  ii. If a person experiences only delusions, whether bizarre or nonbizarre, and has functioning that is not markedly impaired beyond the ramifications of their delusion, consider delusional disorder (full criteria are in DSM-5-TR, pp. 104–106). The criteria include multiple specifiers: erotomanic, grandiose, jealous, persecutory, and somatic. If a person has ever met full criteria for schizophrenia, if the delusions occur during catatonia, if the delusions are due to the physiological effects of a substance or another medical condition, or if the delusions are better explained by another mental disorder, do not make the diagnosis.

  iii. If a person has experienced at least 1 day but less than 1 month of schizophrenia symptoms, consider brief psychotic disorder (full criteria are in DSM-5-TR, pp. 108–109). The person usually experiences an acute onset with emotional turmoil or overwhelming confusion. The person exhibits fewer negative symptoms, experiences less functional impairment, and always experiences an eventual return to their previous level of functioning.

  iv. If a person has experienced at least 1 month but less than 6 months of schizophrenia symptoms, consider schizophreniform disorder (full criteria are in DSM-5-TR, pp. 111–112). This diagnosis should not be used if the disturbance is due to the physiological effects of a substance or another medical condition.

The DSM-5-TR Diagnostic Interview   **81**

v.   If a person who meets criteria for schizophrenia also experiences major mood disturbances—either major depressive episodes or manic episodes—for at least half the time they met criteria for schizophrenia, consider schizoaffective disorder (full criteria are in DSM-5-TR, pp. 121–122). Over the person's lifetime, they must have experienced at least 2 weeks of delusions or hallucinations in the absence of a major mood episode.

vi.   If a substance or medication directly causes delusions and/or hallucinations during substance intoxication or withdrawal, consider substance/medication-induced psychotic disorder (full criteria are in DSM-5-TR, pp. 126–127), while remembering that roughly one-third of people diagnosed with substance-induced psychotic disorder eventually develop schizophrenia spectrum or bipolar disorders when followed longitudinally. The criteria include multiple specifiers for individual substances.

vii.   If another medical condition directly causes the psychotic episode, consider psychotic disorder due to another medical condition (full criteria are in DSM-5-TR, p. 131). This diagnosis should be considered when biological plausibility, temporality, and atypical psychotic symptoms are present. This diagnosis should not be used during an episode of delirium or when the psychotic episode is better explained by another mental disorder.

viii.   If a person experiences psychotic symptoms that cause clinically significant distress or functional impairment without meeting full criteria for another psychotic disorder, consider unspecified schizophrenia spectrum and other psychotic disorder (see DSM-5-TR, p. 138). If you wish to communicate the specific reason a person's symptoms do not meet the criteria, consider other specified schizophrenia spectrum and other psychotic disorder (see DSM-5-TR, p. 138). Examples include persistent auditory hallucinations in the absence of any other feature and delusional symptoms in the partner of an individual with delusional disorder.

Bipolar and Related Disorders

DSM-5-TR pp. 139–175

Screening question: *Have there been times, lasting at least a few days, when you felt really "up" or irritable, and had a lot more energy than usual?*

If yes, ask: *During those times, did you feel this way all day or most of the day? Did those times ever last at least a week or result in your being hospitalized? Did these periods ever cause you significant trouble with your friends or family, at work, or in another setting?*

- If yes, proceed to bipolar I disorder criteria.
- If no, proceed to bipolar II disorder criteria.

1. Bipolar I Disorder

    a. Inclusion: Requires at least <u>three</u> of the following criteria during a manic episode.

        i. Inflated self-esteem or grandiosity: *During that period, did you feel especially confident, as though you could accomplish something extraordinary that you could not have done otherwise?*

        ii. Decreased need for sleep: *During that period, did you notice any change in how much sleep you needed to feel rested? Did you feel rested after less than 3 hours of sleep?*

        iii. More talkative than usual: *During that period, did anyone tell you that you talked more than usual or that it was hard to interrupt you?*

        iv. Flight of ideas: *During that period, were your thoughts racing? Did you have so many ideas you could not keep up with them?*

        v. Distractibility: *During that period, were you having more trouble than usual focusing? Did you find yourself easily distracted?*

        vi. Increased goal-directed activity: *During that period, how did you spend your time? Did you find yourself much more active than usual?*

        vii. Excessive involvement in activities that have a high potential for painful consequences: *During that period, did you engage in activities that were unusual for you? Did you spend money, use substances, or engage in*

> *sexual activities in a way that is unusual for you? Did any of these activities cause trouble for you or someone else?*

b. Exclusion: The occurrence of manic and major depressive episode(s) is not better explained by schizoaffective disorder, schizophrenia, schizophreniform disorder, delusional disorder, or other specified or unspecified schizophrenia spectrum and other psychotic disorder.

c. Exclusion: The episode is not due to the physiological effects of a substance or another medical condition. However, a manic episode that emerges during antidepressant treatment but persists beyond the physiological effect of the treatment meets criteria for the diagnosis.

d. Modifiers

   i. Current (or most recent) episode

- Manic
- Hypomanic
- Depressed
- Unspecified (use when the symptoms but not the duration of the criteria are met)

   ii. Specifiers

- With anxious distress
- With mixed features: Use if at least <u>three</u> of the symptoms of a major depressive episode are present simultaneously.
- With rapid cycling: Use if a patient experienced at least <u>four</u> episodes (manic, hypomanic, or depressive) in the previous 12 months.
- With melancholic features
- With atypical features
- With mood-congruent psychotic features
- With mood-incongruent psychotic features
- With catatonia
- With peripartum onset: Use if the onset of mood symptoms occurs during pregnancy or in the 4 weeks following delivery.
- With seasonal pattern

   iii. Course and severity

- Current or most recent episode manic, hypomanic, depressed, unspecified
    - Mild; Moderate; Severe
    - With psychotic features

- In partial remission; In full remission
- Unspecified

e. Alternatives

  i. If a substance directly causes the episode, including a substance prescribed to treat depression, consider substance/medication-induced bipolar and related disorder (full criteria are in DSM-5-TR, pp. 162–163).

  ii. If another medical condition causes the episode, consider bipolar and related disorder due to another medical condition (full criteria are in DSM-5-TR, p. 166).

2. Bipolar II Disorder

   a. Inclusion: Requires at least <u>three</u> of the following criteria during a hypomanic episode lasting at least 4 days.

      i. Inflated self-esteem or grandiosity: *During that period, did you feel especially confident, as though you could accomplish something extraordinary that you could not have done otherwise?*

      ii. Decreased need for sleep: *During that period, did you notice any change in how much sleep you needed to feel rested? Did you feel rested after less than 3 hours of sleep?*

      iii. More talkative than usual: *During that period, did anyone tell you that you talked more than usual or that it was hard to interrupt you?*

      iv. Flight of ideas: *During that period, were your thoughts racing? Did you have so many ideas you could not keep up with them?*

      v. Distractibility: *During that period, were you having more trouble than usual focusing? Did you find yourself easily distracted?*

      vi. Increased goal-directed activity: *During that period, how did you spend your time? Did you find yourself much more active than usual?*

      vii. Excessive involvement in activities that have a high potential for painful consequences: *During that period, did you engage in activities that were unusual for you? Did you spend money, use substances, or engage in sexual activities in a way that is unusual for you? Did any of these activities cause trouble for anyone?*

b. Exclusion: If there has ever been a manic episode or if the episode is attributable to the physiological effects of a substance/medication, the diagnosis is not given.

c. Exclusion: If the hypomanic episode is better explained by schizoaffective disorder, schizophrenia, schizophreniform disorder, delusional disorder, or other specified or unspecified schizophrenia spectrum and other psychotic disorder, the diagnosis is not given.

d. Modifiers

    i. Specify current or most recent episode

- Hypomanic
- Depressed

    ii. Specifiers

- With anxious distress
- With mixed features: Use if at least <u>three</u> of the symptoms of a major depressive episode are present simultaneously.
- With rapid cycling
- With mood-congruent psychotic features
- With mood-incongruent psychotic features
- With catatonia
- With peripartum onset
- With seasonal pattern
- Unspecified

    iii. Course and severity

- In partial remission
- In full remission
- Unspecified

e. Alternatives

    i. If a person reports 2 or more years of multiple hypomanic and depressive symptoms that never rose to the level of a hypomanic or major depressive episode, consider cyclothymic disorder (full criteria are in DSM-5-TR, pp. 159–160). During the same 2-year period (1 year in children and adolescents), the hypomanic and depressive periods have been present for at least half the time and the individual has not been without the symptoms for more than 2 months at a time. If the symptoms are due to the physiological effects of a substance or another medical condition, the diagnosis is not given.

ii. If a person experiences symptoms characteristic of bipolar disorder that cause clinically significant distress or functional impairment without meeting full criteria for a bipolar disorder, consider unspecified bipolar and related disorder (see DSM-5-TR, p. 169). If you wish to communicate the specific reason a person's symptoms do not meet the criteria, consider other specified bipolar and related disorder (see DSM-5-TR, pp. 168–169). Examples include short-duration hypomanic episodes, short-duration cyclothymia, and hypomanic episode without prior major depressive episode.

Depressive Disorders

DSM-5-TR pp. 177–214

Screening questions: *Have you been feeling sad, empty, or irritable? Have you lost interest in, or do you get less pleasure from, the things you used to enjoy?*

If yes, ask: *Did those times ever last at least 2 weeks? Did these periods ever cause you significant trouble with your friends or family, at work, or in another setting?*

- If yes, proceed to major depressive disorder criteria.
- If a child age 6 years or older says no, ask the irritability screening question, which appears after the alternatives for major depressive disorder below.

1. Major Depressive Disorder, Single and Recurrent Episodes

   a. Inclusion: Requires the presence of at least <u>five</u> of the following symptoms, which must include either depressed mood or loss of interest or pleasure (anhedonia), during the same 2-week episode.

      i. Depressed mood most of the day, nearly every day (already assessed)

      ii. Markedly diminished interest in activities or pleasures (already assessed)

      iii. Significant weight loss or gain: *During that period, did you notice any significant change in your appetite? Did you notice any change in your weight?*

      iv. Insomnia or hypersomnia: *During that period, did you find yourself sleeping more or less than usual? Did you have difficulty getting or staying asleep?*

v. Psychomotor agitation or retardation: *During that period, did anyone tell you that you seemed to move faster or slower than usual?*

vi. Fatigue or loss of energy: *During that period, what was your energy level like? Did anyone tell you that you seemed worn down or less energetic than usual?*

vii. Feelings of worthlessness or excessive guilt: *During that period, did you feel worthless or tremendous regret about current or past events or relationships?*

viii. Diminished concentration: *During that period, were you unable to make decisions or concentrate like you usually do?*

ix. Recurrent thoughts of death or suicide: *During that period, did you think about death more than you usually do? Did you think about hurting yourself or taking your own life? Did you make a plan to suicide?*

b. Exclusion: If there has ever been a manic episode or a hypomanic episode, or the major depressive episode is attributable to the physiological effects of a substance or to another medical condition, the diagnosis is not given.

c. Exclusion: If at least one major depressive episode is better explained by, and superimposed upon, schizo-affective disorder, schizophrenia, schizophreniform disorder, delusional disorder, or other specified or un-specified schizophrenia spectrum and other psychotic disorder, the diagnosis is not given.

d. Modifiers

i. Specifiers
- With anxious distress
- With mixed features: Use if at least <u>three</u> of the symptoms of a manic episode are present simultaneously.
- With melancholic features
- With atypical features (e.g., mood reactivity; weight gain; hypersomnia; leaden paralysis; long pattern of interpersonal rejection sensitivity)
- With mood-congruent psychotic features
- With mood-incongruent psychotic features
- With catatonia
- With peripartum onset (during pregnancy or 4 weeks postpartum)

- With seasonal pattern (onset and remission occur at specific times of the year)

    ii. Course and severity
      - Single episode
      - Recurrent episode

      - In partial remission
      - In full remission

      - Mild
      - Moderate
      - Severe
      - With psychotic features
      - Unspecified

  e. Alternatives

    i. If a person reports experiencing depression for at least 2 years resulting in clinically significant distress or impairment, along with at least <u>two</u> additional symptoms of a major depressive episode, consider persistent depressive disorder (full criteria are in DSM-5-TR, pp. 193–194). If a person experiences 2 continuous months without depressive symptoms, do not give the diagnosis. If the person has ever had a manic or hypomanic episode, do not give the diagnosis. If the disturbance is better explained by a psychotic disorder or is due to the physiological effects of a substance or another medical condition, do not give the diagnosis.

    ii. If a woman describes pronounced mood changes that begin in the week before her menses, improve a few days after the onset of menses, and abate in the week postmenses, consider premenstrual dysphoric disorder (full criteria are in DSM-5-TR, p. 197). The diagnostic criteria include at least <u>one</u> of the following: marked affective lability; marked irritability or interpersonal conflicts; marked depressed mood; and marked anxiety. At least <u>one</u> of the following symptoms must additionally be present (to reach a total of <u>five</u> symptoms when combined with the symptoms above): decreased interest in usual activities; subjective difficulty in concentration; lethargy, easy fatigability, or marked lack of energy; marked change in appetite; hypersomnia or insomnia; sense of being overwhelmed; and physical symptoms such as breast tenderness or swelling, joint/muscle pain, bloating, and weight gain.

iii. If substance intoxication or withdrawal, including from a medication, directly causes a prominent and persistent depressed mood or anhedonia that occurs outside of delirium, consider a substance/medication-induced depressive disorder (full criteria are in DSM-5-TR, pp. 201–202).

iv. If another medical condition directly causes a prominent and persistent depressed mood or anhedonia that occurs outside of delirium, consider a depressive disorder due to another medical condition (full criteria are in DSM-5-TR, p. 206).

v. If a person experiences a depressive episode that causes clinically significant distress or functional impairment without meeting full criteria for a depressive disorder, consider unspecified depressive disorder (see DSM-5-TR, p. 210). If you wish to communicate the specific reason a person's symptoms do not meet the criteria, consider other specified depressive disorder (see DSM-5-TR, pp. 209–210). Examples include recurrent brief depression, short-duration depressive episode, depressive episode with insufficient symptoms, and major depressive disorder superimposed on a psychotic disorder.

vi. If a person experiences symptoms characteristic of a mood disorder causing clinically significant distress or impairment without meeting the full criteria for any specific bipolar or depressive disorder, consider unspecified mood disorder (see DSM-5-TR, p. 210). This diagnosis should be considered when it is difficult to choose, as in acute agitation, between unspecified bipolar and depressive disorder.

Irritability screening question for children: *Do you ever lose your temper, yell, or act out?*

    If yes, ask: *Do you lose your temper every day or every other day? Does your temper or yelling cause trouble at home or school?*

• If yes, proceed to disruptive mood dysregulation disorder criteria.

- If no, seek collateral information from caregivers or proceed to another diagnostic category.
2. Disruptive Mood Dysregulation Disorder
    a. Inclusion: Requires severe recurrent temper outbursts (verbal and/or behavioral) in response to common stressors, averaging at least three per week, for at least 12 months. The outbursts must occur in at least two distinct settings (i.e., home, school, or with peers), be severe in at least one setting, begin before age 10 years, and be characterized by the following <u>three</u> symptoms.
        i. Temper or behavioral outbursts: *When you get upset or lose your temper, what happens? Do you yell? Do you slap, punch, bite, or hit another person? Do you break or destroy things?*
        ii. Disproportionate reaction: *When you get upset or lose your temper, do you know what sets you off? What kinds of things bother you so much that you feel like yelling or hitting?*
        iii. Persistently irritable or angry mood between temper outbursts: *When you are not yelling or upset, how do you feel inside? Do you usually feel grouchy, angry, irritable, or sad?*
    b. Exclusion: These responses must be inconsistent with a child's developmental level.
    c. Exclusion: If the behaviors occur exclusively during an episode of major depressive disorder and are better explained by another mental disorder (e.g., autism spectrum disorder, posttraumatic stress disorder, separation anxiety disorder, persistent depressive disorder), do not make the diagnosis.
    d. Exclusion: If the symptoms are attributable to the physiological effects of a substance or to another medical or neurological condition, do not make the diagnosis.
    e. Exclusion: If a child is currently diagnosed with oppositional defiant disorder, intermittent explosive disorder, or bipolar disorder, do not make the diagnosis.
    f. Alternative: If, during the last year, there was a period lasting more than a day during which the child exhibited abnormally elevated mood and <u>three</u> criteria of a manic episode, consider the possibility of a bipolar disorder (see DSM-5-TR, pp. 139–175).

Anxiety Disorders

DSM-5-TR pp. 215–261

Screening question: *During the past several months, have you frequently been worried about a number of things in your life? Is it hard for you to control or stop your worrying? A panic attack is a sudden surge of intense fear that comes on for no apparent reason, or in situations where you did not expect it to occur. Have you experienced recurrent panic attacks? Do these experiences ever cause you significant trouble with your friends or family, at work, or in another setting?*

    If yes, ask: *Can you identify specific objects, places, or social situations that make you feel very anxious or tearful?*

- If a specific phobia is elicited, proceed to specific phobia disorder criteria.
- If no, first proceed to panic disorder criteria. Then proceed to generalized anxiety disorder criteria.

1. Specific Phobia

   a. Inclusion: Requires that for at least 6 months, a person has experienced marked fear, anxiety, or avoidance as characterized by the following <u>three</u> symptoms.

      i. Specific fear: *Do you fear a specific object or situation such as flying, heights, animals, or something else so much that being exposed to it makes you feel immediately afraid or anxious? What is it?*

      ii. Fear or anxiety provoked by exposure: *When you encounter this, do you experience an immediate sense of fear or anxiety?* For children, ask, *When you encounter this, do you cry, experience tantrums, or hold on to a parent?*

      iii. Avoidance: *Do you find yourself taking steps to avoid this? What are they? When you have to encounter this, do you experience intense fear or anxiety?*

   b. Exclusion: The fear, anxiety, and avoidance are not restricted to objects or situations related to obsessions, reminders of traumatic events, separation from home or attachment figures, or social situations.

   c. Modifiers

      i. Specifiers

         - Descriptive
            - Animal
            - Natural environment

- Blood-injection injury
- Situational
- Other

d. Alternatives

  i. If a person reports developmentally inappropriate and excessive distress when separated from home or a major attachment figure, or expresses persistent worry that his major attachment figure will be harmed or has died, which results in reluctance or refusal to be separated from home or a major attachment figure, consider separation anxiety disorder (full criteria are in DSM-5-TR, p. 217). The onset of this disorder is before age 18. The minimum duration of symptoms necessary to meet the diagnostic criteria is 4 weeks for children and adolescents, but at least 6 months for adults.

  ii. If a person consistently fails to speak in specific social situations for at least 1 month, so that it interferes with educational or occupational achievement, consider selective mutism (full criteria are in DSM-5-TR, p. 222). If the disturbance is due to a lack of knowledge of or comfort with the spoken language, do not give the diagnosis. If the disturbance is better explained by a communication disorder, autism spectrum disorder, or psychotic disorder, do not give the diagnosis.

  iii. If a person reports at least 6 months of marked and disproportionate fear or anxiety about situations such as public transportation, open spaces, being in enclosed spaces, standing in line or being in a crowd, or being outside the home alone, and if these fears cause him to actively avoid these situations, consider agoraphobia (full criteria are in DSM-5-TR, p. 246).

  iv. If a person reports at least 6 months of marked fear or anxiety about, or avoidance of, social situations in which they fear other people will observe or scrutinize them out of proportion to the actual threat posed by these social situations, and the fear, anxiety, or avoidance causes clinically significant distress or impairment, consider social anxiety disorder (full criteria are in DSM-5-TR, pp. 229–230).

2. Panic Disorder

a. Inclusion: Requires recurrent panic attacks, as characterized by at least <u>four</u> of the following symptoms:

i. Palpitations, pounding heart, or accelerated heart rate: *When you experience these sudden surges of intense fear or discomfort, does your heart race or pound?*

ii. Sweating: *During these events, do you find yourself sweating more than usual?*

iii. Trembling or shaking: *During these events, do you shake or develop a tremor?*

iv. Sensations of shortness of breath or smothering: *During these events, do you feel like you are being smothered or cannot catch your breath?*

v. Feelings of choking: *During these events, do you feel as though you are choking, as if something is blocking your throat?*

vi. Chest pain or discomfort: *During these events, do you feel intense pain or discomfort in your chest?*

vii. Nausea or abdominal distress: *During these events, do you feel sick to your stomach or like you need to vomit?*

viii. Feeling dizzy, unsteady, light-headed, or faint: *During these events, do you feel dizzy, light-headed, or like you may faint?*

ix. Chills or heat sensations: *During these events, do you feel very cold and shiver, or do you feel intensely hot?*

x. Paresthesias: *During these events, do you feel numbness or tingling?*

xi. Derealization or depersonalization: *During these events, do you feel like people or places that are familiar to you are unreal, or that you are so detached from your body that it is like you are standing outside your body or watching yourself?*

xii. Fear of losing control: *During these events, do you fear you may be losing control, or even "going crazy"?*

xiii. Fear of dying: *During these events, do you fear you may be dying?*

b. Inclusion: At least <u>one</u> panic attack is followed by at least 1 month of at least one of the following symptoms:

i. Persistent worry about consequences: *Are you persistently concerned or worried about additional panic attacks? Are you persistently concerned or worried that these attacks mean you are having a heart attack, losing control, or "going crazy"?*

ii. Maladaptive change to avoid attacks: *Have you made significant maladaptive changes in your behavior, like avoiding unfamiliar situations or exercise, in order to avoid attacks?*

c. Exclusion: If the disturbance is better explained by another mental disorder or is attributable to the physiological effects of a substance/medication or another medical condition, do not make the diagnosis.

d. Alternatives

i. If a person reports panic attacks as described above but neither experiences persistent worry about consequences nor makes significant maladaptive behavioral changes to avoid panic attacks, consider using the panic attack specifier (see DSM-5-TR, p. 242). The panic attack specifier can be used with other anxiety disorders, as well as with bipolar, depressive, traumatic, and substance use disorders.

3. Generalized Anxiety Disorder

a. Inclusion: Requires excessive anxiety and worry that is difficult to control, occurring more days than not for at least 6 months, about a number of events or activities, associated with at least <u>three</u> of the following symptoms.

i. Restlessness: *When you think about events or activities that make you anxious or worried, do you often feel restless, on edge, or keyed up?*

ii. Easily fatigued: *Do you find that you often tire or fatigue easily?*

iii. Difficulty concentrating: *When you are anxious or worried, do you often found it hard to concentrate or find that your mind goes blank?*

iv. Irritability: *When you are anxious or worried, do you often feel irritable or easily annoyed?*

v. Muscle tension: *When you are anxious or worried, do you often experience muscle tightness or tension?*

vi. Sleep disturbance: *Do you find it difficult to fall asleep or stay asleep, or experience restless and unsatisfying sleep?*

b. Exclusion: If the anxiety and worry are better explained by another mental disorder or are attributable to the physiological effect of a substance/medication or another medical condition, do not make the diagnosis.

c. Alternatives

i. If a substance directly causes the episode, through exposure, intoxication, or withdrawal, including a medication prescribed to treat a mental disorder, consider a substance/medication-induced anxiety disorder (full criteria are in DSM-5-TR, pp. 255–256).

ii. If another medical condition directly causes the anxiety and worry, consider an anxiety disorder due to another medical condition (full criteria are in DSM-5-TR, pp. 258–259).

iii. If a person experiences symptoms characteristic of an anxiety disorder that cause clinically significant distress or functional impairment without meeting full criteria for another anxiety disorder, consider unspecified anxiety disorder (see DSM-5-TR, p. 261). If you wish to communicate the specific reason a person's symptoms do not meet the criteria for a specific anxiety disorder, consider other specified anxiety disorder (see DSM-5-TR, p. 261). Examples include *khyâl* (wind attacks), *ataque de nervios* (attack of nerves), and generalized anxiety not occurring more days than not.

Obsessive-Compulsive and Related Disorders

DSM-5-TR pp. 263–294

Screening questions: *Do you frequently experience intrusive and unwanted images, thoughts, or urges? Are there any physical acts that you feel like you have to do in order to avoid or reduce the distress associated with these images, thoughts, or urges?*

If yes, ask: *Do these experiences or behaviors ever cause you significant trouble with your friends or family, at work, or in another setting?*

• If yes, proceed to obsessive-compulsive disorder criteria.
• If no, proceed to body-focused repetitive behavior screening questions, which follow the obsessive-compulsive disorder section below.

1. Obsessive-Compulsive Disorder

   a. Inclusion: Requires the presence of obsessive thoughts, compulsive behaviors, or both, as manifested by the following symptoms.

      i. Obsessive thoughts (as defined by both questions): *When you experience these intrusive and unwanted im-*

ages, thoughts, or urges, do they make you really anxious or distressed? Do you have to work hard to ignore or suppress these kinds of thoughts?

ii. Compulsive behaviors (as defined by both questions): *Some people try to reverse intrusive ideas by repeatedly performing some kind of action such as hand washing or lock checking, or by a mental act such as counting, praying, or silently repeating words. Do you do something like that? Do you think that doing so will reduce your distress or prevent something you dread from occurring?*

b. Inclusion: The obsessions or compulsions are time-consuming (e.g., take more than 1 hour per day) or cause clinically significant distress or impairment.

c. Exclusions

i. If the obsessions or compulsions are better explained by another mental disorder, do not make the diagnosis. If the obsessive-compulsive symptoms are due to the physiological effects of a substance or another medical condition, do not make the diagnosis.

ii. If a person reports that their intrusive images, thoughts, or urges are pleasurable, they do not meet the criteria for an obsessive-compulsive disorder. Instead, consider substance use disorders, personality disorders, and paraphilic disorders.

iii. If a person reports intrusive images, thoughts, or urges centered on more real-world concerns, consider an anxiety disorder.

d. Modifiers

i. Specifiers

• Insight

• With good or fair insight: Use if a person recognizes that his beliefs are definitely or probably untrue.

• With poor insight: Use if a person thinks his beliefs are probably true.

• With absent insight/delusional beliefs: Use if a person is completely convinced his beliefs are true.

• Tic-related: Use if a person meets criteria for a current or lifetime chronic tic disorder.

e. Alternatives

    i. If a person reports intrusive images, thoughts, or urges centered on their body image, consider body dysmorphic disorder (full criteria are in DSM-5-TR, pp. 271–272). The criteria include preoccupation with perceived defects in physical appearance beyond concern about weight or body fat in a person with an eating disorder, repetitive behaviors or mental acts in response to concern about appearance, and clinically significant distress or impairments because of the preoccupation.

    ii. If a person reports persistent difficulty in parting with possessions regardless of their value, consider hoarding disorder (full criteria are in DSM-5-TR, p. 277). The criteria include strong urges to save items, distress associated with discarding items, and the accumulation of a large number of possessions that clutter the home or workplace to the extent that it can no longer be used for its intended function.

    iii. If a substance directly causes the condition, including a substance prescribed to treat depression, consider substance/medication-induced obsessive-compulsive and related disorder (full criteria are in DSM-5-TR, pp. 287–289).

    iv. If another medical condition directly causes the episode, consider obsessive-compulsive and related disorder due to another medical condition (full criteria are in DSM-5-TR, p. 291).

    v. If a person experiences symptoms characteristic of an obsessive-compulsive and related disorder that cause clinically significant distress or functional impairment without meeting full criteria for another obsessive-compulsive and related disorder, consider unspecified obsessive-compulsive and related disorder (see DSM-5-TR, p. 294). If you wish to communicate the specific reason a person's symptoms do not meet the criteria for a specific obsessive-compulsive and related disorder, consider other specified obsessive-compulsive and related disorder (see DSM-5-TR, pp. 293–294). Examples include body dysmorphic–like disorder with actual flaws, body dysmorphic–like disorder without repetitive behaviors, body-focused repetitive behavior disorder, obsessional jealousy disorder, olfactory reference disorder, *Shubo-kyofu*, and *koro*.

2. Body-Focused Repetitive Behaviors

   a. Inclusion: DSM-5-TR includes two conditions, trichotillomania (hair-pulling disorder) and excoriation (skin-picking) disorder, with nearly identical criteria. Either diagnosis requires the presence of <u>all three</u> of the following symptoms.

      i. Behavior: *Do you frequently pull your hair or pick at your skin so much that it causes hair loss or skin lesions?*
      ii. Repeated attempts to change: *Have you repeatedly tried to decrease or stop this behavior?*
      iii. Impairment: *Does this behavior cause you to feel ashamed or out of control? Do you avoid work or social settings because of these behaviors?*

   b. Alternatives

      i. If the behavior is attributable to another medical condition or to substance use, or is better explained by another mental disorder, you should not diagnose either trichotillomania or excoriation disorder.

Trauma- and Stressor-Related Disorders

DSM-5-TR pp. 295–328

Screening questions: *What is the worst thing that has ever happened to you? Have you ever experienced or witnessed an event in which you were seriously injured or your life was in danger, or you thought you were going to be seriously injured or endangered?*

If yes, ask: *Do you think about or reexperience these events? Does thinking about these experiences ever cause significant trouble with your friends or family, at work, or in another setting?*

- If yes, proceed to posttraumatic stress disorder criteria.
- If a child says no but his family or caregivers report disturbances in his primary attachments, proceed to reactive attachment disorder criteria.

1. Posttraumatic Stress Disorder

   a. Inclusion: Requires exposure to actual or threatened death, serious injury, or sexual violation in at least one of the following ways: direct experience; in-person witnessing; learning of actual or threatened death, serious injury, or sexual violation of a close family member or friend; repeated or extreme exposure to aversive details of traumatic event(s). In addition, a person must experience at least one of the following intrusion symptoms for at least 1 month after the traumatic experience.

    i. Memories: *After that experience, did you ever experience intrusive memories of the experience when you did not want to think about it?* For children, repetitive reenactment through play qualifies. *Do you repeatedly reenact that experience with your toys or dolls or when playing?*

    ii. Dreams: *Did you have recurrent, distressing dreams related to the experience?* For children, frightening dreams without recognizable content qualifies. *Do you frequently have very frightening dreams that you cannot recall or describe?*

    iii. Flashbacks: *After that experience, did you ever feel like it was happening to you again, like in a flashback where the event is happening again?* For children, this may be observed in their play.

    iv. Exposure distress: *When you are around people, places, and objects that remind you of that experience, do you feel intense or prolonged distress?*

    v. Physiological reactions: *When you think about or are around people, places, and objects that remind you of that experience, do you have distressing physical responses?*

b. Inclusion: In addition, a person must experience at least <u>one</u> of the following avoidance symptoms for at least 1 month after the traumatic experience.

    i. Internal reminders: *Do you work hard to avoid thoughts, feelings, or physical sensations that bring up memories of this experience?*

    ii. External reminders: *Do you work hard to avoid people, places, and objects that bring up memories of this experience?*

c. Inclusion: In addition, a person must experience at least <u>two</u> of the following negative symptoms for at least 1 month.

    i. Impaired memory: *Do you have trouble remembering important parts of the experience?*

    ii. Negative self-image: *Do you frequently think negative thoughts about yourself, other people, or the world?*

   iii. Blame: *Do you frequently blame yourself or others for your experience, even when you know that you or they were not responsible?*

   iv. Negative emotional state: *Do you stay down, angry, ashamed, or fearful most of the time?*

   v. Decreased participation: *Are you much less interested in activities in which you used to participate?*

   vi. Detachment: *Do you feel detached or estranged from the people in your life because of this experience?*

   vii. Inability to experience positive emotions: *Do you find that you cannot feel happy, loved, or satisfied? Do you feel numb, or like you cannot love?*

d. Inclusion: In addition, a person must experience at least <u>two</u> of the following arousal behaviors.

   i. Irritable or aggressive: *Do you often act very grumpy or even get verbally or physically aggressive?*

   ii. Reckless: *Do you often act reckless or self-destructive?*

   iii. Hypervigilance: *Are you always on edge or keyed up?*

   iv. Exaggerated startle: *Do you startle easily?*

   v. Impaired concentration: *Do you often have trouble concentrating on a task or problem?*

   vi. Sleep disturbance: *Do you often have difficulty falling asleep or staying asleep, or do you often wake up without feeling rested?*

e. Exclusion: The episode is not directly caused by a substance or by another medical condition.

f. Modifiers

   i. Subtypes

     • With dissociative symptoms, either depersonalization or derealization

     • Posttraumatic stress disorder for children 6 years and younger: Reserved for children under age 6 years who experienced trauma themselves, witnessed trauma, or learned of trauma experienced by a parent or other caregiver (full criteria are in DSM-5-TR, pp. 303–304).

   ii. Specifiers

     • With delayed expression: Use if a person does not exhibit all the diagnostic criteria until at least 6 months after the traumatic experience.

g. Alternatives

    i. If the episode lasts less than 1 month and the experience occurred within the past month, and the person experiences at least <u>nine</u> of the posttraumatic symptoms described above, consider acute stress disorder (full criteria are in DSM-5-TR, pp. 313–315).

    ii. If the episode began within 3 months of the experience and a person does not meet the symptomatic and behavioral criteria for posttraumatic stress disorder or a prolonged grief disorder, consider an adjustment disorder (full criteria are in DSM-5-TR, pp. 319–320). The criteria include marked distress disproportionate to an acute stressor, either traumatic or nontraumatic, and significant impairment in function.

    iii. If a person experiences symptoms characteristic of a trauma- and stressor-related disorder that cause clinically significant distress or functional impairment without meeting full criteria for one of the named disorders, consider unspecified trauma- and stressor-related disorder (see DSM-5-TR, p. 328). If you wish to communicate the specific reason a person's symptoms do not meet the criteria for a specific trauma- and stressor-related disorder, consider other specified trauma- and stressor-related disorder (see DSM-5-TR, pp. 327–328). Examples include persistent complex bereavement disorder and adjustment-like disorder with delayed onset of symptoms that occur more than 3 months after the stressor.

    iv. If a person experiences persistent grief after the death of someone they were close to, consider prolonged grief disorder (see DSM-5-TR, pp. 322–323). The death must have occurred at least 6 months ago for a child or adolescent to meet criteria and at least 12 months ago for an adult. For the criteria to be met, a person must experience, nearly daily, intense yearning/longing for the deceased or preoccupation with thoughts or memories of the deceased that exceeds expected cultural or social norms. For the criteria to be met, the person must have been experiencing three or more of these symptoms nearly daily for the last month: identity disruption; marked sense of disbelief about the death; avoidance of reminders that the person is dead; intense emotional pain; difficulty reintegrating into activities and relationships; emotional numbness; feeling that life is meaningless; and intense loneliness.

2. Reactive Attachment Disorder

   a. Inclusion: Requires that a child experience extremes of insufficient care, before age 5 years, that result in <u>both</u> of the following behaviors.

      i. Rare or minimal comfort seeking: *When you are feeling really angry, upset, or sad, do you rarely seek comfort or consolation from other people?*

      ii. Rare or minimal response to comfort: *When you are feeling really angry, upset, or sad and somebody says or does something nice for you, do you find that you only feel a little better?*

   b. Inclusion: Requires the persistent experience of at least <u>two</u> of the following states.

      i. Relative lack of social and emotional responsiveness to others: *When you interact with other people, do you usually respond with very little feeling or emotion?*

      ii. Limited positive affect: *Do you usually find it hard to be excited, self-assured, and cheerful?*

      iii. Episodes of unexplained irritability, sadness, or fearfulness, which are evident during nonthreatening interactions with caregivers: *Do you often have episodes where you become irritable, sad, or afraid with an adult caregiver who does not pose a threat to you?*

   c. Inclusion: Requires the persistent experience of at least <u>one</u> of the following states.

      i. Social neglect or deprivation in the form of persistent lack of having basic emotional needs for comfort, stimulation, and affection met

      ii. Repeated changes of primary caregivers that limit opportunities to form stable attachments

      iii. Rearing in unusual settings that severely limit opportunities to form selective attachments

   d. Exclusions

      i. If a child does not have a developmental age of at least 9 months, do not make the diagnosis.

ii. If a child meets criteria for autism spectrum disorder, do not make the diagnosis.

e. Modifiers

i. Specifiers

- Persistent: Use when the disorder is present for more than 12 months.

ii. Severity: Specified severe when a child meets all symptoms of the disorder, with each symptom manifesting in relatively high levels

f. Alternative: If a young child who has experienced extremes of insufficient care exhibits profoundly disturbed externalizing behavior, consider disinhibited social engagement disorder (full criteria are in DSM-5-TR, pp. 298–299). The criteria include at least two of the following symptoms: reduced reticence with unfamiliar adults, overly familiar verbal or physical behavior, diminished checking back with an adult caregiver after venturing away, and a willingness to go off with an unfamiliar adult with minimal or reduced hesitation.

Dissociative Disorders

DSM-5-TR pp. 329–348

Screening questions: *Everyone has trouble remembering things sometimes, but do you ever lose time, forget important details about yourself, or find evidence that you took part in events you cannot recall? Do you ever feel like people or places that are familiar to you are unreal, or that you are so detached from your body that it is like you are standing outside your body or watching yourself?*

If yes, ask: *Did these experiences ever cause you significant trouble with your friends or family, at work, or in another setting?*

- If amnesia predominates, proceed to dissociative amnesia criteria.
- If depersonalization or derealization predominates, proceed to depersonalization/derealization disorder criteria.

1. Dissociative Amnesia

a. Inclusion: Requires the presence of inability to recall important autobiographical information beyond ordinary forgetting, most often manifested by at least <u>one</u> of the following symptoms.

    i. Localized or selective amnesia: *Do you find yourself unable to recall a specific event or events in your life, especially events that were really stressful or even traumatic?*

    ii. Generalized amnesia: *Do you find yourself unable to freely recall important moments in your life history or details of your very identity?*

b. Exclusions

    i. If the disturbance is better accounted for by dissociative identity disorder, posttraumatic stress disorder, acute stress disorder, somatic symptom disorder, or major or mild neurocognitive disorder, do not make the diagnosis.

    ii. If the disturbance is due to the physiological effects of a substance or a neurological or other medical condition, do not make the diagnosis.

c. Modifiers

    i. Specifiers

      • With dissociative fugue: Use when a person engages in purposeful travel or bewildered wandering for which they have amnesia.

d. Alternatives

    i. If a person reports a disruption of identity, characterized by two or more distinct personality states or an experience of possession, that causes clinically significant distress and functional impairment, consider dissociative identity disorder (full criteria are in DSM-5-TR, p. 330). The criteria include recurrent gaps in recall that are inconsistent with ordinary forgetting and dissociative experiences that are not a normal part of a broadly accepted cultural or religious practice and that are not attributable to the physiological effects of a substance or another medical condition.

2. Depersonalization/Derealization Disorder

a. Inclusion: Requires at least <u>one</u> of the following manifestations.

    i. Depersonalization: *Do you frequently have experiences of unreality or detachment—like you are an outside ob-*

server of your mind, thoughts, feelings, sensations, body, or whole self?

  ii. Derealization: *Do you frequently have experiences of unreality or detachment from your surroundings—like you often experience people or places as unfamiliar, unreal, dreamlike, or visually distorted?*

b. Inclusion: Requires intact reality testing. *During these experiences, can you distinguish these experiences from actual events—what is occurring outside of you?*

c. Exclusions

  i. If the disturbance is due to the physiological effects of a substance or a neurological or other medical condition, do not make the diagnosis.

  ii. If depersonalization or derealization occurs exclusively as symptoms of or during the course of another mental disorder, do not make the diagnosis.

d. Alternatives

  i. If a person is experiencing a disorder whose most prominent symptoms are amnestic but does not meet the criteria for a specific disorder, consider other specified or unspecified dissociative disorder (see DSM-5-TR, pp. 347–348). Examples include subthreshold dissociative disturbances in identity and memory, chronic and recurrent syndromes of mixed dissociative symptoms, identity disturbances in individuals subjected to prolonged periods of intense coercive persuasion, acute reactions to stressful situations, acute psychotic states intermixed with dissociative symptoms in a person who does not meet criteria for delirium or a psychotic disorder, and dissociative trance.

Somatic Symptom and Related Disorders

DSM-5-TR pp. 349–370

Screening questions: *Do you worry about your physical health more than most people? Do you get sick more often than most people?* **If yes, ask:** *Do these experiences significantly affect your daily life?*

If yes, ask: *Which is worse for you, worrying about the symptoms you experience or worrying about your health and the possibility that you are sick?*

- If worry about symptoms predominates, proceed to somatic symptom disorder criteria.
- If worry about being ill or sick predominates, proceed to illness anxiety disorder criteria.

1. Somatic Symptom Disorder

   a. Inclusion: Requires at least <u>one</u> somatic symptom that is distressing. *Do you experience unexplained symptoms that cause you to feel anxious or distressed? Do these symptoms significantly disrupt your daily life?*

   b. Inclusion: Requires at least <u>one</u> of the following thoughts, feelings, or behaviors, typically for at least 6 months.

      i. Disproportionate thoughts: *Do you find yourself persistently thinking about your health concerns and how serious they are?*

      ii. Persistently high level of anxiety: *Do you persistently feel a high level of anxiety or worry about your health concerns?*

      iii. Excessive investment: *Do you find yourself investing a lot more time and energy into your health concerns than you would like to?*

   c. Modifiers

      i. Specifiers
         - With predominant pain
         - Persistent

      ii. Severity
         - Mild: One of the symptoms specified in (b) above
         - Moderate: Two or more of the symptoms specified in (b) above
         - Severe: Two or more of the symptoms specified in (b) above plus multiple somatic complaints (or one very severe somatic symptom)

   d. Alternatives

      i. If a person is focused on the loss of bodily function rather than on the distress a particular symptom causes, consider functional neurological symptom disorder (conversion disorder) (full criteria are in DSM-5-TR, pp. 360–361). The criteria for this disorder include symptoms of altered voluntary motor or sensory function, clinical evidence that these symptoms are clearly incompatible with recognized neurological or medical conditions, and significant impairment in social or occupational functioning. When possible, specify the symptom type using available specifiers, including with weakness or paralysis, with abnormal movement, with swallowing symptoms, with speech symptoms, with attacks or seizures, and with special sensory symptoms.

ii. If a person has a documented medical condition other than a mental disorder, but behavioral or psychological factors adversely affect the course of their medical condition by delaying recovery, decrease adherence, significantly increase health risks, or influence the underlying pathophysiology, consider psychological factors affecting other medical conditions (full criteria are in DSM-5-TR, pp. 364–365).

iii. If a person falsifies physical or psychological signs or symptoms, or induces injury or disease to deceptively present themselves to others as ill, impaired, or injured, consider factitious disorder imposed on self (full criteria are in DSM-5-TR, p. 367). For the criteria to be met, the person needs to exhibit these behaviors even in the absence of obvious external rewards. The symptoms cannot be better accounted for by another mental disorder such as a psychotic disorder.

iv. If a person falsifies physical or psychological signs or symptoms, or induces injury or disease, to deceptively present someone else to others as ill, impaired, or injured, consider factitious disorder imposed on another (full criteria are in DSM-5-TR, p. 367). The diagnosis is assigned to the perpetrator rather than the victim, and for the criteria to be met, the behavior needs to occur even in the absence of obvious external rewards, and not be better explained by another mental disorder such as a psychotic disorder.

2. Illness Anxiety Disorder

a. Inclusion: Requires all of the following symptoms for at least 6 months and the absence of somatic symptoms.

i. Preoccupation: *Do you find yourself preoccupied about having or acquiring a serious illness?*

ii. Anxiety: *Do you feel a high level of anxiety or alarm about having or acquiring a serious illness?*

iii. Associated behaviors: *Have these worries affected your behavior? Some people find themselves frequently checking their body for signs of illness, reading about illness all the time, or avoiding persons, places, or objects to ward off illness. Do you find yourself doing any things like that?*

b. Exclusion: If a person's symptoms are better explained by another mental disorder, do not make the diagnosis.

c. Modifiers

i. Subtypes

  • Care-seeking
  • Care-avoidant

ii. Course

  • Transient

d. Alternatives

i. If a person endorses symptoms characteristic of a somatic symptom disorder that cause clinically significant distress or impairment without meeting the full criteria for a specific somatic symptom and related disorder, consider unspecified somatic symptom and related disorder (see DSM-5-TR, p. 370). If you wish to communicate specific reasons that full criteria are not met, consider other specified somatic symptom and related disorder (see DSM-5-TR, p. 370). Examples of other presentations in the other specified category include brief somatic symptom disorder, brief illness anxiety disorder, illness anxiety disorder without excessive health-related behaviors or maladaptive avoidance, and pseudocyesis.

Feeding and Eating Disorders

DSM-5-TR pp. 371–397

Screening questions: *What do you think of your appearance? Do you ever restrict or avoid particular foods so much that it negatively affects your health or weight?*

If yes, ask: *When you consider yourself, is the shape or weight of your body one of the most important things about you?*

- If yes, proceed to anorexia nervosa criteria.
- If no, proceed to avoidant/restrictive food intake disorder criteria.

1. Anorexia Nervosa

    a. Inclusion: Requires the presence of <u>all three</u> of the following features.

        i. Energy restriction leading to significantly low body weight adjusted for age, developmental trajectory, physical health, and sex: *Have you limited the food you eat to achieve a low body weight? What was the least you ever weighed? What do you weigh now?*

        ii. Fear of weight gain or behavior interfering with weight gain: *Have you ever experienced intense fear of gaining weight or becoming fat? Has there ever been a time when you were already at a low weight and still did things to interfere with gaining weight?*

        iii. Disturbance in self-perceived weight or shape: *How do you experience the weight and shape of your body? Are there particular parts of your body that you frequently evaluate or measure? How do you think having a significantly low body weight will affect your physical health?*

    b. Modifiers

        i. Subtypes

            - Restricting type: Use when a person reports no recurrent episodes of bingeing or purging in the last 3 months.
            - Binge-eating/purging type: Use when a person reports recurrent episodes of bingeing or purging in the last 3 months.

        ii. Specifiers

            - In partial remission
            - In full remission

        iii. Severity (based on body mass index [BMI])

            - Mild: BMI ≥ 17 kg/m^2
            - Moderate: BMI 16–16.99 kg/m^2
            - Severe: BMI 15–15.99 kg/m^2
            - Extreme: BMI < 15 kg/m^2

c. Alternatives

    i. If a person reports recurrent binge eating, recurrent inappropriate compensatory behaviors to prevent weight gain (e.g., misuse of laxatives or other medications, self-induced vomiting, excessive exercise), and self-image unduly influenced by the shape or weight of his body, consider bulimia nervosa (full criteria are in DSM-5-TR, pp. 387–388). The diagnosis requires that binge eating and compensatory behaviors both occur, on average, at least once a week for 3 months. The diagnosis cannot be made if bingeing and compensating behaviors occur only during episodes of anorexia nervosa.

    ii. If a person has recurrent episodes of binge eating characterized <u>both</u> by eating an amount of food that is definitely larger than most people would eat in a similar period of time under similar circumstances and by a sense of lack of control over eating during the episode, consider binge-eating disorder (full criteria are in DSM-5-TR, pp. 392–393). Binge-eating episodes are associated with at least <u>three</u> of the following: eating much more rapidly than normal, eating until feeling uncomfortably full, eating large amounts of food when not feeling physically hungry, eating alone because of feeling embarrassed by how much one is eating, and feeling disgusted with oneself, depressed, or very guilty after overeating. For the diagnosis to be made, a person must experience marked distress regarding the binge eating, and binge eating must occur, on average, at least once a week for 3 months. Finally, the binge eating cannot occur exclusively during the course of anorexia nervosa or bulimia nervosa.

2. Avoidant/Restrictive Food Intake Disorder

    a. Inclusion: Requires significant disturbance in eating or feeding as manifested by at least <u>one</u> of the following.

        i. Significant weight loss: *Do you avoid certain foods or restrict what you eat to the extent that it has seriously affected your weight? Have you experienced a significant weight loss as a result?* For children: *Do you avoid or restrict food to the extent that you have not grown at the expected rate?*

ii. Significant nutritional deficiency: *Do you avoid or restrict food to the extent that it has negatively affected your health, as in experiencing a significant nutritional deficiency?*

iii. Dependence on enteral feeding or oral supplements: *Have you avoided or restricted food to the extent that you depend on tube feedings or oral supplements to maintain nutrition?*

iv. Marked interference with psychosocial functioning: *Has avoiding or restricting food impaired your ability to participate in your usual social activities or made it hard to form or sustain relationships? Can you eat with other people or participate in social activities when food is present?*

b. Exclusion: If the eating disturbance is better explained by lack of available food (e.g., food insecurity) or by an associated culturally sanctioned practice (e.g., religious fasting), or by eating practices related to a disturbance in body image, do not make the diagnosis.

c. Exclusion: If the eating disturbance occurs exclusively during anorexia nervosa or bulimia nervosa, is attributable to another medical condition, or is better explained by another mental disorder, do not make the diagnosis.

d. Modifiers

  i. Specifiers

   • In remission

e. Alternatives

  i. If a person persistently eats nonnutritive nonfood substances over a period of at least 1 month, consider pica (see DSM-5-TR, pp. 371–372). The eating of nonnutritive, nonfood substances must be inappropriate to their developmental stage and must not be part of a culturally supported or socially normative practice.

  ii. If a person repeatedly regurgitates food over a period of at least 1 month, consider rumination disorder (full criteria are in DSM-5-TR, p. 374). For this diagnosis, the regurgitation cannot occur as the result of an associated gastrointestinal or other medical condition, and the regurgitation cannot occur exclusively during the course of anorexia nervosa, bulimia nervosa, binge-eating disorder, or avoidant/restrictive food intake disorder.

iii. If a person has an atypical, mixed, or subthreshold disturbance in his eating and feeding, or if you lack sufficient information to make a more specific diagnosis, consider other specified or unspecified feeding and eating disorder (see DSM-5-TR, pp. 396–397). DSM-5-TR also allows the use of this category for specific syndromes that are not formally included, such as atypical anorexia nervosa, night eating syndrome, and purging disorder.

Elimination Disorders

DSM-5-TR pp. 399–405

Screening question: *Have you repeatedly passed urine or feces onto your clothing, your bed, the floor, or another place where urine or feces are not usually deposited?*

- If passing urine, proceed to enuresis criteria.
- If passing feces, proceed to encopresis criteria.

1. Enuresis

    a. Inclusion: In addition to the intentional or involuntary repeated voiding of urine into one's bed or clothes, requires the following frequency.

        i. Occurs at least twice a week for at least 3 consecutive months: *Has this occurred at least twice a week? Has it also occurred for 3 months in a row?*

    b. Exclusions

        i. If a person is younger than age 5 years, or the equivalent developmental age, do not make the diagnosis.

        ii. If the behavior is due to the physiological effects of a substance or another medical condition through a mechanism other than constipation, do not make the diagnosis.

    c. Modifiers

        i. Nocturnal only

        ii. Diurnal only: either urge incontinence (sudden urge symptoms) or voiding postponement (conscious deferral of micturition urges)

        iii. Nocturnal and diurnal

2. Encopresis

   a. Inclusion: In addition to the intentional or involuntary repeated voiding of feces into inappropriate places (e.g., clothing, floor), requires the following frequency.

      i. Occurs at least monthly for at least 3 consecutive months: *Has this occurred at least once a month? Has it also occurred for 3 months in a row?*

   b. Exclusions

      i. If a person is younger than 4 years, or the equivalent developmental age, do not make the diagnosis.

      ii. If the behavior is attributable to the physiological effects of a substance or another medical condition through a mechanism other than constipation, do not make the diagnosis.

   c. Modifiers

      i. With constipation and overflow incontinence
      ii. Without constipation and overflow incontinence

   d. Alternatives

      i. If a person experiences symptoms characteristic of an elimination disorder that cause clinically significant distress or impairment without meeting the full criteria for an elimination disorder, consider unspecified elimination disorder (see DSM-5-TR, p. 405). If you wish to communicate specific reasons that full criteria are not met, consider other specified elimination disorder (see DSM-5-TR, p. 405).

Sleep-Wake Disorders

DSM-5-TR pp. 407–476

Screening questions: *Is your sleep often inadequate or of poor quality? Alternatively, do you often experience excessive sleepiness? Do you frequently experience an irrepressible need to sleep or experience sudden lapses into sleep? Have you, or a sleeping partner, noticed any unusual behaviors while you sleep? Have you, or a sleeping partner, noticed that you stop breathing or gasp for air while sleeping?*

• If dissatisfaction with sleep quantity or quality predominates, proceed to insomnia disorder criteria.

- If excessive sleep predominates, proceed to hypersomnolence disorder criteria.
- If an irrespressible need to sleep or sudden lapses into sleep predominate, proceed to narcolepsy criteria.
- If unusual sleep behaviors (parasomnias) predominate, proceed to restless legs syndrome criteria.
- If sleep breathing problems predominate, proceed to obstructive sleep apnea hypopnea criteria.

1. Insomnia Disorder

    a. Inclusion: Requires dissatisfaction with sleep quantity or quality, at least 3 nights per week, for at least 3 months, as manifested by at least <u>one</u> of the following symptoms.

        i. Difficulty initiating sleep: *Do you often have trouble getting to sleep? For children: Do you often have trouble getting to sleep without the help of a parent or someone else?*
        ii. Difficulty maintaining sleep: *After you get to sleep, do you frequently awaken when you do not want to wake up? Do you often have difficulty returning to sleep after these awakenings? For children: If you wake up when you wanted to be asleep, do you need the help of a parent or someone else to get back to sleep?*
        iii. Early-morning awakening: *Do you often wake up earlier than you intended and find yourself unable to return to sleep?*

    b. Exclusion: The sleep difficulty must occur despite adequate opportunity for sleep.
    c. Exclusion: If the insomnia is better explained by or occurs exclusively during the course of another sleep-wake disorder, is attributable to the physiological effects of a substance, or is better explained by a co-existing mental disorder or medical condition, do not make the diagnosis.
    d. Modifiers

        i. Specifiers

            - With non–sleep disorder mental comorbidity, including substance use disorders
            - With other medical comorbidity
            - With other sleep disorder

ii. Course
- Episodic
- Recurrent
- Persistent

e. Alternatives

i. If a person experiences a persistent or recurrent pattern of sleep disruption leading to excessive sleepiness, insomnia, or both, and this disruption is primarily due to an alteration of the circadian system or to a misalignment between the endogenous circadian rhythm and the sleep-wake schedule required by the person's physical environment or social/professional schedule, consider a circadian rhythm sleep-wake disorder (full criteria, along with multiple subtypes, are in DSM-5-TR, pp. 443–451). The sleep disturbance must cause clinically significant distress or functional impairment.

ii. If substance use, intoxication, or withdrawal is etiologically related to insomnia, consider substance/medication-induced sleep disorder, insomnia type (full criteria, along with multiple subtypes, are in DSM-5-TR, pp. 468–469). The disturbance cannot be better accounted for by delirium, a non-substance-induced sleep disorder, or the sleep symptoms usually associated with an intoxication or withdrawal syndrome. The disorder must cause significant distress or functional impairment.

iii. If a person meets all criteria for an insomnia disorder but the duration has been less than 3 months, consider unspecified insomnia disorder (see DSM-5-TR, p. 475). The diagnosis is reserved for insomnia symptoms that produce significant distress or functional impairment. If you wish to communicate the reason a person's symptoms do not meet the full criteria for a specific sleep disorder, consider other specified insomnia disorder (see DSM-5-TR, p. 475).

2. Hypersomnolence Disorder

a. Inclusion: Requires excessive sleepiness at least three times per week for at least 3 months, despite a main sleep period lasting at least 7 hours, that causes significant distress or functional impairment. The hypersomnolence is manifested by at least <u>one</u> of the following symptoms.

   i. Recurrent periods of sleep: *Do you often have several periods of sleep within the same day?*
   ii. Prolonged nonrestorative sleep episode: *Do you often have a main sleep episode, lasting at least 9 hours, that is not refreshing or restorative?*
   iii. Sleep inertia: *Do you often have difficulty being fully awake? After an awakening, do you often feel groggy or notice that you have trouble engaging in tasks or activities that would otherwise be simple for you?*

b. Exclusion: If the hypersomnia occurs exclusively during the course of another sleep disorder, is better accounted for by another sleep disorder, or is attributable to the physiological effects of a substance, do not make the diagnosis.

c. Modifiers

   i. Specifiers

- With mental disorder, including substance use disorders
- With mental condition
- With another sleep disorder

   ii. Course

- Acute: Use when duration is less than 1 month.
- Subacute: Use when duration is 1–3 months.
- Persistent: Use when duration is greater than 3 months.

   iii. Severity

- Mild: Difficulty maintaining daytime alertness 1–2 days/week
- Moderate: Difficulty maintaining daytime alertness 3–4 days/week
- Severe: Difficulty maintaining daytime alertness 5–7 days/week

d. Alternative: If substance use, intoxication, or withdrawal is etiologically related to daytime sleepiness, consider substance/medication-induced sleep disorder, daytime sleepiness type (full criteria, along with multiple subtypes, are in DSM-5-TR, pp. 468–469). The disturbance cannot be better accounted for by delirium, a non-substance-induced sleep disorder, or the sleep symptoms usually associated with an intoxication or withdrawal syndrome. The disorder must cause significant distress or functional impairment.

3. Narcolepsy

   a. Inclusion: Requires periods of an irrepressible need to sleep or lapsing into sleep, at least three times per week over the past 3 months, along with at least <u>one</u> of the following.

      i. Episodes of cataplexy:

         - For a person with long-standing narcolepsy: *At least a few times a month, do you find that after you laugh or joke, you suddenly and briefly lose muscle tone on both sides of your body but remain conscious?*
         - For children or a person with ≤6 months of narcolepsy: *At least a few times a month, do you find that all of a sudden you grimace, open your mouth wide and thrust out your tongue, or lose muscle tone throughout your body, without any obvious emotional trigger?*

      ii. Hypocretin deficiency: Measured using cerebrospinal fluid hypocretin-1 (CSF-1) immunoreactivity values.

      iii. Nocturnal sleep polysomnography showing rapid eye movement (REM) sleep latency ≤15 minutes or a multiple sleep latency test showing mean sleep latency ≤8 minutes and ≥ sleep-onset REM periods.

   b. Modifiers

      i. Subtypes

         - Narcolepsy with cataplexy or hypocretin deficiency
         - Narcolepsy without cataplexy and either without hypocretin deficiency or hypocretin unmeasured
         - Narcolepsy with cataplexy or hypocretin deficiency due to a medical condition
         - Narcolepsy without cataplexy and without hypocretin deficiency due to a medical condition

      ii. Severity

         - Mild: Need for naps only once or twice per day. Sleep disturbance, if present, is mild. Cataplexy, when present, occurs less than once per week.

- Moderate: Need for multiple naps daily. Sleep may be moderately disturbed. Cataplexy, when present, occurs daily or every few days.
- Severe: Nearly constant sleepiness. Often highly disturbed nocturnal sleep (i.e., excessive movements, vivid dreaming). Cataplexy, when present, is drug-resistant, with multiple attacks daily.

4. Obstructive Sleep Apnea Hypopnea

   a. Inclusion: Requires repeated episodes of upper airway obstruction during sleep. There must be polysomnographic evidence of at least five obstructive apneas or hypopneas per hour of sleep, and <u>either</u> of the following symptoms.

      i. Nocturnal breathing disturbances: *Do you often disturb your sleeping partner with snoring, snorting, gasping for air, or breathing pauses during sleep?*

      ii. Daytime sleepiness, fatigue, or nonrestorative sleep: *When you have an opportunity to get sleep, do you still wake up the next day feeling exhausted, sleepy, or fatigued?*

   b. Inclusion: Alternatively, the diagnosis can be made by polysomnographic evidence of 15 or more obstructive apneas or hypopneas per hour of sleep regardless of accompanying symptoms.

   c. Modifiers

      i. Severity

         - Mild: Use when a person's apnea hypopnea index is less than 15.
         - Moderate: Use when a person's apnea hypopnea index is between 15 and 30.
         - Severe: Use when a person's apnea hypopnea index is greater than 30.

   d. Alternatives

      i. If a person demonstrates five or more central apneas per hour of sleep during polysomnographic examination, and this disturbance is not better accounted for by another current sleep disorder, consider central sleep apnea (full criteria are in DSM-5-TR, pp. 435–436).

      ii. If a person demonstrates episodes of shallow breathing associated with arterial oxygen desaturation and/or elevated carbon dioxide levels during poly-somnographic examination, and this disturbance is not better accounted for by another current sleep disorder, consider sleep-related hypoventilation (full criteria are in DSM-5-TR, pp. 439–440). This disorder is most commonly associated with medical or neurological disorders, obesity, medication use, or substance use disorders.

5. Restless Legs Syndrome

   a. Inclusion: Requires an urge to move the legs, usually accompanied by or in response to uncomfortable and unpleasant sensations in the legs, at least three times per week for at least 3 months, as manifested by <u>all</u> of the following symptoms.

      i. Urge to move legs: *While you are asleep, do you often experience uncomfortable or unpleasant sensations in the legs? Do you often experience an urge to move your legs?*

      ii. Relieved with movement: *Are these partially or completely relieved by moving your legs?*

      iii. Nocturnal worsening: *What times of day do you most experience the urge to move your legs? Is it worse in the evening or at night than during the day?*

   b. Exclusions

      i. If these symptoms are attributable to a medical condition or to the physiological effects of a substance, or are better explained by another mental disorder or behavioral condition, do not make the diagnosis.

   c. Alternatives

      i. If a person experiences recurrent episodes of incomplete awakening from sleep in which they experience an abrupt and terrifying awakening (sleep terror) or they rise from bed and walk about (sleepwalking), usually during the first third of the major sleep episode, consider non–rapid eye movement sleep arousal disorders (full criteria are in DSM-5-TR, p. 452). When experiencing an episode, the person experiences little to no dream imagery. The person experiences amnesia for the episode and is relatively unresponsive to efforts of other people.

      ii. If a person repeatedly experiences extremely dysphoric and well-remembered dreams and rapidly becomes alert and oriented upon awakening from these dysphoric dreams, consider nightmare disorder (full criteria are in DSM-5-TR, p. 457). The dream disturbance, or the sleep disturbance produced by awakening from the nightmare, causes clinically significant distress or functional impairment. The dysphoric dreams do not occur exclusively during another mental disorder or are not a physiological effect of a substance/medication or another medical condition.

iii. If a person repeatedly experiences episodes of arousal from sleep associated with vocalization and/or complex motor behaviors sufficient to result in injury to themselves or their bed partner, consider rapid eye movement sleep behavior disorder (full criteria are in DSM-5-TR, p. 461). These behaviors arise during REM sleep and typically occur more than 90 minutes after sleep onset. Upon awakening, the person is fully awake, alert, and oriented. The diagnosis requires <u>either</u> polysomnographic evidence of REM sleep disturbance or evidence that the behaviors are injurious, potentially injurious, or disruptive.

iv. If substance or medication use, intoxication, or withdrawal is etiologically related to a parasomnia, consider substance/medication-induced sleep disorder, parasomnia type (full criteria are in DSM-5-TR, pp. 468–469). The disturbance cannot be better accounted for by delirium, a non-substance-induced sleep disorder, or the sleep symptoms usually associated with an intoxication or withdrawal syndrome. The disorder must cause significant distress or functional impairment.

v. If a person has an atypical, mixed, or subthreshold disturbance in sleeping and waking, consider other specified or unspecified sleep-wake disorder (see DSM-5-TR, p. 476).

Sexual Dysfunctions

DSM-5-TR pp. 477–509

Screening question: *Have you been less interested in sex than usual or experienced difficulties in sexual performance?*

If yes, ask: *Have these experiences lasted at least 6 months and caused you significant distress or impairment?*

- If disinterest in sex predominates, proceed to female sexual interest/arousal disorder criteria for women or male hypoactive sexual desire disorder for men.
- If difficulties in sexual performance predominate, proceed to female orgasmic disorder for women or erectile disorder for men.

1. Erectile Disorder
   a. Inclusion: Requires the presence of at least <u>one</u> of the following symptoms on almost all or all occasions of sexual activity, for at least 6 months.
      i. Difficult to obtain: *During sexual activity, have you noticed a marked difficulty in obtaining an erection?*
      ii. Difficult to maintain: *Do you have a marked difficulty in maintaining an erection until the completion of sexual activity?*
      iii. Decrease in rigidity: *Have you experienced a decrease in the rigidity of your erections severe enough that it interferes with sexual activity?*
   b. Exclusion: If a man has sexual dysfunction that is better accounted for by a nonsexual mental disorder, severe relationship distress, or another significant stressor, or is attributable to the effects of a substance/medication or another medical condition, do not make the diagnosis.
   c. Modifiers
      i. Subtypes
         - Generalized: Not limited to certain types of stimulation, situations, or partners
         - Situational: Only occurs with certain types of stimulation, situations, or partners
      ii. Specifiers
         - Lifelong: Disturbance has been present since the individual became sexually active.
         - Acquired: Disturbance began after a period of relatively normal sexual function.
      iii. Severity
         - Mild: Evidence of mild distress over the symptoms
         - Moderate: Evidence of moderate distress over the symptoms

- Severe: Evidence of severe or extreme distress over the symptoms

d. Alternatives

i. If a man reports that during almost all or all partnered sexual experiences over at least the last 6 months, he experienced an undesired and marked infrequency or delay in ejaculation, consider delayed ejaculation (full criteria are in DSM-5-TR, pp. 478–479). If the symptoms are better explained by a nonsexual mental disorder or severe relationship distress, do not give the diagnosis.

ii. If a man reports that he ejaculated within approximately 1 minute following vaginal penetration during almost all or all partnered experiences over at least the last 6 months, without wishing to do so, consider premature (early) ejaculation (full criteria are in DSM-5-TR, pp. 501–502).

2. Female Orgasmic Disorder

a. Inclusion: Requires the presence of <u>one</u> of the following symptoms during all or almost all sexual experiences, for at least 6 months.

i. Delayed, absent, or infrequent orgasms: *Does it take you much longer than usual to achieve orgasm, or do you rarely or never experience an orgasm?*

ii. Reduced intensity of orgasms: *Have you noticed the intensity of your orgasms is markedly reduced?*

b. Exclusion: If a woman has sexual dysfunction that is better explained by a nonsexual mental disorder, severe relationship distress, or another significant stressor, or is attributable to the effects of a substance/medication or another medical condition, do not make the diagnosis.

c. Modifiers

i. Subtypes

- Generalized: Not limited to certain types of stimulation, situations, or partners
- Situational: Only occurs with certain types of stimulation, situations, or partners

ii. Specifiers

- Lifelong: Disturbance has been present since the individual became sexually active

- Acquired: Disturbance began after a period of relatively normal sexual function
- Never experienced an orgasm under any situation

iii. Severity
- Mild: Evidence of mild distress over the symptoms
- Moderate: Evidence of moderate distress over the symptoms
- Severe: Evidence of severe or extreme distress over the symptoms

d. Alternatives

i. If a woman reports at least 6 months of marked difficulty having vaginal intercourse, marked vulvovaginal or pelvic pain during vaginal intercourse, marked fear or anxiety either about vulvovaginal or pelvic pain or vaginal penetration, or marked tensing or tightening of the pelvic floor muscles during attempted vaginal penetration, consider genito-pelvic pain/penetration disorder (full criteria are in DSM-5-TR, pp. 493–494).

3. Female Sexual Interest/Arousal Disorder

a. Inclusion: Requires at least 6 months without, or with reduced, sexual interest or arousal as manifested by at least <u>three</u> of the following symptoms.

i. Absent/reduced sexual interest: *Have you noticed that the intensity or frequency of your interest in sexual activity is absent or markedly reduced?*

ii. Absent/reduced sexual thoughts: *Have you noticed that the intensity or frequency of your sexual thoughts or fantasies is absent or markedly reduced?*

iii. No/reduced sexual initiation: *Have you noticed that the intensity or frequency with which you initiate sexual activity, or respond to a partner's initiation, is absent or markedly reduced?*

iv. Absent/reduced sexual excitement/pleasure: *When you engage in sexual encounters, have you noticed that almost all of the time, your experience of sexual excitement or pleasure is absent or markedly reduced?*

v. Absent/reduced sexual response: *Have you noticed that the intensity or frequency with which you experi-*

ence sexual interest in response to erotic signals is absent or markedly reduced?*

    vi. Absent/reduced sexual sensations: *When you engage in sexual encounters, have you noticed that almost all of the time, the intensity or frequency with which you experience genital or nongenital sensation is absent or markedly reduced?*

b. Exclusion: If a woman has sexual dysfunction that is better accounted for by a nonsexual mental disorder, severe relationship distress, or another significant stressor, or is attributable to the effects of a substance/medication or another medical condition, do not make the diagnosis.

c. Modifiers

    i. Subtypes

- Generalized: Not limited to certain types of stimulation, situations, or partners
- Situational: Only occurs with certain types of stimulation, situations, or partners

- Lifelong: Disturbance has been present since the individual became sexually active
- Acquired: Disturbance began after a period of relatively normal sexual function

    ii. Severity

- Mild: Evidence of mild distress over the symptoms
- Moderate: Evidence of moderate distress over the symptoms
- Severe: Evidence of severe or extreme distress over the symptoms

d. Alternatives

    i. If a woman has a clinically significant disturbance in sexual function directly associated with the use or discontinuation of a substance or medication, consider a substance/medication-induced sexual dysfunction (full criteria are in DSM-5-TR, pp. 504–506).

    ii. If a woman has a sexual dysfunction, but the symptoms do not meet the threshold for another sexual dysfunction diagnosis, the etiology is uncertain, or there is insufficient information to diagnose a current sexual dysfunction, consider unspecified sexual dysfunction (see DSM-5-TR, p. 509). If you wish to communicate the specific reason a person's symptoms do not meet full criteria, consider other specified sexual dysfunction (see DSM-5-TR, p. 509).

4. Male Hypoactive Sexual Desire Disorder

   a. Inclusion: Requires persistently or recurrently deficient (or absent) sexual thoughts or fantasies and desires for at least 6 months.

      i. Absent sexual thoughts: *Have you noticed that the intensity or frequency of your sexual thoughts, desires, or fantasies is absent or markedly reduced?*

   b. Exclusion: If a man has sexual dysfunction that is better accounted for by a nonsexual mental disorder, severe relationship distress, or another significant stressor, or is attributable to the effects of a substance/medication or another medical condition, do not make the diagnosis.

   c. Modifiers

      i. Subtypes

         • Generalized: Not limited to certain types of stimulation, situations, or partners
         • Situational: Only occurs with certain types of stimulation, situations, or partners
         • Lifelong: Disturbance has been present since the individual became sexually active
         • Acquired: Disturbance began after a period of relatively normal sexual function

      ii. Severity

         • Mild: Evidence of mild distress over the symptoms
         • Moderate: Evidence of moderate distress over the symptoms
         • Severe: Evidence of severe or extreme distress over the symptoms

   d. Alternatives

      i. If a man has a clinically significant disturbance in sexual function directly associated with the use or discontinuation of a substance or medication, consider a substance/medication-induced sexual dysfunction (full criteria are in DSM-5-TR, pp. 504–506).

ii. If a man has a sexual dysfunction but the symptoms do not meet the threshold for another sexual dysfunction diagnosis, the etiology is uncertain, or there is insufficient information to diagnose a current sexual dysfunction, consider unspecified sexual dysfunction (see DSM-5-TR, p. 509). If you wish to communicate the specific reason a person's symptoms do not meet full criteria, consider other specified sexual dysfunction (see DSM-5-TR, p. 509).

Gender Dysphoria

DSM-5-TR pp. 511–520

Screening question: *Are you really uncomfortable with your birth-assigned gender?*

If yes, ask: *Has this discomfort lasted at least 6 months and gotten to the point where you really feel like your given gender is incongruent with your gender identity? Does this discomfort cause significant trouble with your friends or family, at work, or in another setting?*

- If a child or his parent says yes, proceed to gender dysphoria in children.
- If an adolescent or adult says yes, proceed to gender dysphoria in adolescents and adults.

1. Gender Dysphoria in Children

   a. Inclusion: Requires at least <u>six</u> of the following manifestations (one of which must be a strong desire to be of the other gender), of at least 6 months' duration.

      i. Desire to be of other gender: *Have you experienced a strong desire to be of a gender other than your given gender? Do you insist that people treat you as a member of a gender other than your given gender?*

      ii. Cross-dressing: *Do you have a strong preference for clothes usually associated with a gender other than your given gender?*

      iii. Cross-gender fantasy: *When you play fantasy games, do you have a strong preference for cross-gender roles?*

      iv. Cross-gender play: *When you play, do you have a strong preference for toys or activities that most people associate with the other gender?*

    v. Cross-gender playmates: *Do you have a strong prefer-ence for friends of the other gender?*

   vi. Rejection of toys, games, and activities typically associated with given gender: *Do you strongly reject the toys, games, and activities typically associated with your given gender?*

 vii. Dislike of anatomy: *Do you have a strong dislike for your sexual anatomy?*

viii. Desire to have other sex characteristics: *Have you experienced a strong desire for the primary or secondary sex characteristics that match your experience of gender?*

  b. Specifiers

- With a disorder/difference of sex development

2. Gender Dysphoria in Adolescents and Adults

  a. Inclusion: Requires at least <u>two</u> of the following manifestations, of at least 6 months' duration.

    i. Incongruence: *Have you experienced a profound sense that your primary or secondary sex characteristics do not match your gender identity?*

   ii. Desire to change: *Have you experienced a profound desire to change your primary or secondary sex characteristics because they do not match your gender identity?*

  iii. Desire to have sex characteristics of other gender: *Have you experienced a strong desire for the primary or secondary sex characteristics that match your experience of gender?*

  iv. Desire to be of other gender: *Have you experienced a strong desire to be of a gender other than your given gender?*

   v. Desire to be treated as other gender: *Have you experienced a strong desire to be treated as a gender other than your given gender?*

  vi. Conviction that one has feelings of other gender: *Have you experienced a strong conviction that your typical feelings and reactions are those of the gender other than your given gender?*

  b. Modifiers

    i. Specifiers

- With a disorder/difference of sex development
- Posttransition: The individual has transitioned to full-time living in the experienced gender (with or without legalization of gender change)

and has undergone (or is preparing to have) at least one gender-affirming medical procedure or treatment regimen

  c. Alternatives

   i. If a person experiences symptoms characteristic of gender dysphoria that cause clinically significant distress or impairment without meeting the full criteria for gender dysphoria, consider unspecified gender dysphoria (see DSM-5-TR, p. 520). If you wish to communicate the specific reason a person's symptoms do not meet full criteria, consider other specified gender dysphoria (see DSM-5-TR, p. 520)

Disruptive, Impulse-Control, and Conduct Disorders

DSM-5-TR pp. 521–541

Screening questions: *Do you often have times when you become so upset that you make or even act upon verbal or physical threats to hurt other people, animals, or property? Have you ever been aggressive to people and animals, destroyed property, deceived other people, or stolen things?*

  If yes, ask: *Have these behaviors ever caused you significant trouble with your friends or family, at school or work, with the authorities, or in another setting?*

• If recurrent behavioral outbursts predominate, proceed to intermittent explosive disorder criteria.
• If recurrent rule breaking predominates, proceed to conduct disorder criteria.

1. Intermittent Explosive Disorder

  a. Inclusion: Requires recurrent behavioral outbursts in which the person does not control his aggressive impulses, as manifested by <u>either</u> of the following.

   i. Verbal or physical aggression: *Over the past 3 months, have you had impulsive outbursts in which you were verbally or physically aggressive toward other people, animals, or property? Have these outbursts occurred, on average, at least twice weekly?*

ii. Three behavioral outbursts involving damage to or destruction of property and/or physical assault: *Over the last 12 months, have you lost control of your behavior three or more times and destroyed property or assaulted other people?*

b. Inclusion: Also requires all <u>three</u> of the following.

   i. Magnitude of aggressiveness is disproportionate to any provocation or psychosocial stressor: *Looking back at these outbursts, can you identify any events or stressors associated with them? Was your response much more aggressive or extreme than these events or stressors?*

   ii. Recurrent outbursts are neither premeditated nor in pursuit of a tangible objective: *When you had these outbursts, did they happen when you were feeling angry or impulsive? Did the outburst occur without a clear goal like obtaining money or intimidating someone?*

   iii. Outbursts cause marked personal distress, impair function, or are associated with financial or legal consequences: *How do these outbursts affect how you feel about yourself and how you get along with friends, family, and other people in your life? Have you ever suffered financial or legal consequences because of your outbursts?*

c. Exclusions

   i. If the recurrent aggressive outbursts are fully explained by another mental disorder, or attributable to another medical condition or to the physiological effects of a substance/medication, do not make the diagnosis.

   ii. For children: If aggressive behavior occurs only in the context of an adjustment disorder, do not make the diagnosis. If chronological age, or equivalent developmental level, is less than 6 years, do not make the diagnosis.

2. Conduct Disorder

a. Inclusion: Requires a repetitive and persistent pattern of behavior in which the basic rights of others or major age-appropriate societal norms or rules are violated, as manifested by the presence of at least <u>three</u> of the following in the past 12 months and at least <u>one</u> of the following in the past 6 months.

i. Often bullies, threatens, or intimidates others: *Do you often bully, threaten, or intimidate other people?*

ii. Often initiates physical fights: *Do you often start physical fights?*

iii. Has used a weapon that can cause serious physical harm to others: *Have you used a weapon that could cause serious harm to someone else, such as a bat, brick, broken bottle, knife, or gun?*

iv. Has been physically cruel to people: *Have you caused physical pain or suffering in other people?*

v. Has been physically cruel to animals: *Have you caused physical pain or suffering in animals?*

vi. Has stolen while confronting a victim: *Have you forcibly taken or stolen something from someone while the person was present?*

vii. Has forced someone into sexual activity: *Have you forced someone into sexual activity?*

viii. Has deliberately engaged in fire setting with the intention of causing serious damage: *Have you set fires in order to cause serious damage to a person, animal, or property?*

ix. Has deliberately destroyed others' property: *Have you deliberately destroyed someone else's belongings?*

x. Has broken into someone else's house, building, or car: *Have you broken into someone else's house, building, or car?*

xi. Often lies to obtain goods or favors or to avoid obligations: *Do you often lie to get out of work or to get things you want?*

xii. Has stolen items of nontrivial value without confronting a victim: *Have you taken or stolen something valuable from someone when the person was not present?*

xiii. Often stays out at night despite parental prohibitions, beginning before age 13: *Before the age of 13, did you have a curfew, a time after which you had to be at home, that you often violated by staying out later than you were supposed to?*

xiv. Has run away from home overnight at least twice while living in the parental or parental surrogate home (or once without returning for a lengthy period): *Have you ever run away from home? How many times? Did you ever run away from home and not return for a long time?*

xv. Is often truant from school, beginning before age 13: *Before the age of 13, did you often cut class or skip school?*

b. Exclusion: If a person is 18 years or older and meets the criteria for antisocial personality disorder, do not make the diagnosis.

c. Modifiers

  i. Subtypes

   • Childhood-onset type: Use when at least one criterion symptom begins before age 10 years.
   • Adolescent-onset type: Use when no criterion symptoms are present before age 10 years.
   • Unspecified onset: Use when the age at onset is unknown.

  ii. Specifiers

   • With limited prosocial emotions: Use for a person who persistently exhibits at least two of the following characteristics: lack of remorse or guilt, callous lack of empathy, lack of concern about performance, and shallow or deficient affect. To meet criteria, these characteristics must be displayed in multiple relationships and settings over at least 12 months. These characteristics reflect a person's typical pattern of interpersonal and emotional functioning and not just occasional occurrences in some situations.

  iii. Severity

   • Mild: Few, if any, conduct problems beyond those required for diagnosis, and relatively minor harm to others
   • Moderate: Intermediate number of conduct problems and intermediate harm to others.
   • Severe: Many conduct problems beyond those required for diagnosis, or considerable harm to others

d. Alternatives

  i. If a person exhibits at least 6 months of a frequent and persistent pattern of angry and irritable mood along with defiant or vindictive behavior, consider oppositional defiant disorder (full criteria, along with specifiers, are in DSM-5-TR, pp. 522–523). The pattern is manifested by at least four of the following: frequent loss of temper, being touchy or easily annoyed by others, being angry and resentful, arguing with authority figures, actively defying or refusing to comply with the requests or rules of authority figures, deliberately annoying people, blaming others for one's mistakes or misbehaviors, and at least two episodes of being spiteful or vindictive within the past 6 months. The behaviors must also cause clinically significant impairment and cannot occur exclusively during the course of a psychotic, substance use, depressive, or bipolar disorder, and the criteria for disruptive mood dysregulation disorder cannot be met. In addition, it is important to consider the persistence and frequency of these behaviors in relation to a person's developmental stage. For children younger than age 5, the behavior must occur on most days for at least 6 months. For children age 5 years or older, the behavior must occur at least once a week for at least 6 months.

ii. If a person reports deliberate and purposeful fire-setting on at least two occasions, consider pyromania (full criteria are in DSM-5-TR, p. 537). The diagnosis requires tension or affective arousal before the fire setting, fascination with fire, and pleasure or relief when setting or witnessing fires. If the fire setting is done for monetary gain, to improve a living situation, to express an ideology, to conceal criminal activity, for vengeance, or in response to a hallucination, do not make the diagnosis. If the fire setting is better explained by intellectual developmental disorder, conduct disorder, mania, or antisocial personality disorder, do not make the diagnosis.

iii. If a person repeatedly fails to resist impulses to steal objects that are not needed for his personal use or their monetary value, consider kleptomania (full criteria are in DSM-5-TR, p. 539). The diagnosis requires tension or affective arousal before the theft, and pleasure or relief at the time of the theft. If the stealing is done out of anger or vengeance, or in response to a hallucination, do not make the diagnosis. If the stealing is better explained by conduct disorder, mania, or antisocial personality disorder, do not make the diagnosis.

iv. If a person exhibits symptoms characteristic of a disruptive, impulse-control, and conduct disorder that cause clinically significant distress or impairment without meeting the full criteria for a diagnosis named above, consider unspecified disruptive, impulse-control, and conduct disorder (see DSM-5-TR, p. 541). If you wish to communicate the specific reason a person does not meet the full criteria, consider other specified disruptive, impulse-control, and conduct disorder (see DSM-5-TR, p. 541).

Substance-Related and Addictive Disorders

DSM-5-TR pp. 543–665

Screening questions: *How often do you drink alcohol? On an average day when you have at least one drink, how many total drinks do you end up having? Have you had any problems as a result of drinking? When you stop drinking, do you go through withdrawal?*

Repeat for illicit and prescription drugs; begin by asking: *Have you ever experimented with drugs?*

After asking about drugs, ask: *Do you bet, wager, or gamble in a way that interferes with your life?*

If yes, ask: *Did these experiences ever cause you significant trouble with your friends or family, at work, or in another setting?*

- If a person reports problems with substance use, proceed to the substance use disorder criteria for the particular substance.
- If a person presents with substance intoxication, proceed to the substance intoxication criteria for the particular substance.
- If a person reports problems with substance withdrawal, proceed to the substance withdrawal criteria for the particular substance.
- If a person reports problems with gambling, proceed to gambling disorder criteria.

1. Alcohol Use Disorder

    a. Inclusion: Requires a problematic pattern of alcohol use leading to clinically significant impairment or distress as manifested by at least <u>two</u> of the following in a 12-month period.

i. Drinking more alcohol over a longer period than intended: *When you drink, do you find that you drink more, or for a longer time, than you planned to?*

ii. Persistent desire or unsuccessful effort to reduce alcohol use: *Do you want to cut back or stop drinking? Have you ever tried and failed to cut back or stop drinking?*

iii. Great deal of time spent: *Do you spend a great deal of your time obtaining alcohol, drinking alcohol, or recovering from your alcohol use?*

iv. Cravings: *Do you experience strong desires or cravings to drink alcohol?*

v. Failure to fulfill major role obligations: *Have you repeatedly failed to fulfill major obligations at work, home, or school because of your alcohol use?*

vi. Continued use despite awareness of interpersonal or social problems: *Do you drink alcohol even though you suspect, or even know, that it creates or worsens interpersonal or social problems?*

vii. Giving up activities for alcohol: *Are there important social, occupational, or recreational activities that you have given up or reduced because of your alcohol use?*

viii. Use in hazardous situations: *Have you repeatedly used alcohol in situations in which it was physically hazardous, such as driving a car or operating a machine while intoxicated?*

ix. Continued use despite awareness of physical or psychological problems: *Do you drink alcohol even though you suspect, or even know, that it creates or worsens problems with your mind and body?*

x. Tolerance as manifested by <u>either</u> of the following.

- Markedly increased amounts: *Do you find that in order to get intoxicated or achieve the desired effect of drinking, you need to consume much more alcohol than you used to?*
- Markedly diminished effects: *If you drink the same amount of alcohol as you used to, do you find that it has a lot less effect on you than it used to?*

xi. Withdrawal as manifested by <u>either</u> of the following.

- Characteristic alcohol withdrawal syndrome: *When you stop drinking, do you undergo withdrawal?*
- The same or a closely related substance is taken to relieve or avoid withdrawal symptoms: *Have*

you ever drunk alcohol or taken another substance to prevent alcohol withdrawal?

    b. Modifiers

        i. Specifiers

- In early remission
- In sustained remission
- In a controlled environment

       ii. Severity

- Mild: Use when two or three criteria are present.
- Moderate: Use when four or five criteria are present.
- Severe: Use when six or more criteria are present.

    c. Alternatives

        i. If a person received more than minimal exposure to alcohol at any time during gestation and experiences neurocognitive impairment, impaired self-regulation, and deficits in adaptive functioning, consider neurobehavioral disorder associated with prenatal alcohol exposure (an other specified neurodevelopmental disorder; see DSM-5-TR, p. 99). The diagnosis requires onset of symptoms before age 18 years and clinically significant distress or functional impairment.

       ii. If a person experiences problems associated with the use of alcohol that are not classifiable as alcohol use disorder, intoxication, withdrawal, intoxication delirium, withdrawal delirium, or as an alcohol-induced neurocognitive disorder, psychotic disorder, bipolar disorder, depressive disorder, anxiety disorder, sexual dysfunction, or sleep disorder, consider unspecified alcohol-related disorder (see DSM-5-TR, p. 568).

2. Alcohol Intoxication

    a. Inclusion: Requires at least <u>one</u> of the following signs or symptoms shortly after alcohol use.

        i. Slurred speech
       ii. Incoordination
      iii. Unsteady gait
      iv. Nystagmus
       v. Impairment in attention or memory
      vi. Stupor or coma

b. Inclusion: Requires clinically significant problematic behavioral or psychological changes. *Since you began this episode of drinking, have you observed any significant changes in your behavior, mood, or judgment? Have you done problematic things, or thought problematic thoughts, that you would not have if you were sober?*

c. Exclusion: If the symptoms are attributable to another medical condition or are better explained by another mental disorder, including intoxication with another substance, do not make the diagnosis.

3. Alcohol Withdrawal

a. Inclusion: Requires at least <u>two</u> of the following symptoms, developing within several hours to a few days of ceasing (or reducing) alcohol use that has been heavy and prolonged.

   i. Autonomic hyperactivity

   ii. Increased hand tremor

   iii. Insomnia: *Over the last couple of days, have you found it more difficult than usual to get to sleep and to stay asleep?*

   iv. Nausea or vomiting: *Over the last couple of days, have you felt sick to your stomach, felt nauseated, or even vomited?*

   v. Transient visual, tactile, or auditory hallucinations or illusions: *Over the last couple of days, have you had any experiences where you worried that your mind was playing tricks on you, such as seeing, hearing, or feeling things that other people could not?*

   vi. Psychomotor agitation

   vii. Anxiety: *Over the last couple of days, have you felt more worried or anxious than usual?*

   viii. Generalized tonic-clonic seizures

b. Exclusion: If the symptoms are attributable to another medical condition or better explained by another mental disorder, including intoxication with or withdrawal from another substance, do not make the diagnosis.

c. Modifiers

   i. Specifiers

      • With perceptual disturbances: Use when hallucinations occur with intact reality testing or when auditory, visual, or tactile illusions occur in the absence of delirium.

4. Caffeine Intoxication

   a. Inclusion: Requires clinically significant problematic behavioral or psychological changes shortly after caffeine ingestion, usually in excess of 250 mg (e.g., 2–3 cups of brewed coffee), as manifested by at least <u>five</u> of the following signs.

      i. Restlessness: *Over the last several hours, have you felt less able to remain at rest than usual?*

      ii. Nervousness: *Over the last several hours, have you felt more jittery or nervous than usual?*

      iii. Excitement: *Over the last several hours, have you felt more excited than usual?*

      iv. Insomnia: *Over the last several hours, if you tried to sleep, did you find it more difficult to get to sleep or stay asleep than usual?*

      v. Flushed face

      vi. Diuresis: *Over the last several hours, have you urinated more often or a greater amount than usual?*

      vii. Gastrointestinal disturbance: *Over the last several hours, have you experienced an upset stomach, nausea, vomiting, or diarrhea?*

      viii. Muscle twitching: *Over the last several hours, have you noticed your muscles twitching more than usual?*

      ix. Rambling flow of thought and speech: *Over the last several hours, have you or anyone else noticed that your thoughts or speech has been long-winded or even confused?*

      x. Tachycardia or cardiac arrhythmia

      xi. Periods of inexhaustibility: *Over the last several hours, have you felt like you had so much energy it could not be used up?*

      xii. Psychomotor agitation

   b. Exclusion: If the symptoms are attributable to another medical condition or better explained by another mental disorder, including intoxication with another substance, do not make the diagnosis.

   c. Alternative: If a person experiences problems associated with the use of caffeine that are not classifiable as caffeine intoxication, caffeine withdrawal, caffeine-induced anxiety disorder, or caffeine-induced sleep disorder, consider unspecified caffeine-related disorder (see DSM-5-TR, p. 574).

5. Caffeine Withdrawal

   a. Inclusion: Requires at least <u>three</u> of the following symptoms, developing within 24 hours of ceasing (or reducing) caffeine use that has been prolonged.

      i. Headache: *Over the last day, have you had any headaches?*
      ii. Marked fatigue or drowsiness: *Over the last day, have you felt extremely tired or sleepy?*
      iii. Dysphoric or depressed mood or irritability: *Over the last day, have you felt more down, depressed, or irritable than usual?*
      iv. Difficulty concentrating: *Over the last day, have you had difficulty staying focused on a task or activity?*
      v. Flu-like symptoms: *Over the last day, have you experienced flu-like symptoms, nausea, vomiting, or muscle pain or stiffness?*

   b. Exclusion: If the symptoms are attributable to another medical condition or are better explained by another mental disorder, including intoxication with or withdrawal from another substance, do not make the diagnosis.

6. Cannabis Use Disorder

   a. Inclusion: Requires a problematic pattern of cannabis use leading to clinically significant impairment or distress as manifested by at least <u>two</u> of the following in a 12-month period.

      i. Consuming more cannabis over a longer period than intended: *When you use cannabis, do you find that you use more, or for a longer time, than you planned to?*
      ii. Persistent desire or unsuccessful effort to reduce cannabis use: *Do you want to cut back or stop using cannabis? Have you ever tried and failed to cut back or stop?*
      iii. Great deal of time spent: *Do you spend a great deal of your time obtaining cannabis, using cannabis, or recovering from your cannabis use?*
      iv. Cravings: *Do you experience strong desires or cravings to use cannabis?*
      v. Failure to fulfill major role obligations: *Have you repeatedly failed to fulfill major obligations at work, home, or school because of your cannabis use?*
      vi. Continued use despite awareness of interpersonal or social problems: *Do you use cannabis even though*

you suspect, or even know, that it creates or worsens interpersonal or social problems?

vii. Giving up activities for cannabis: *Are there important social, occupational, or recreational activities that you have given up or reduced because of your cannabis use?*

viii. Use in hazardous situations: *Have you repeatedly used cannabis in situations in which it was physically hazardous, such as driving a car or operating a machine while intoxicated?*

ix. Continued use despite awareness of physical or psychological problems: *Do you use cannabis even though you suspect, or even know, that it creates or worsens problems with your mind and body?*

x. Tolerance as manifested by <u>either</u> of the following.

- Markedly increased amounts: *Do you find that in order to get high or achieve the desired effect of using cannabis, you need to smoke or ingest much more cannabis than you used to?*
- Markedly diminished effects: *If you use the same amount of cannabis as you used to, do you find that it has a lot less effect on you than it used to?*

xi. Withdrawal as manifested by <u>either</u> of the following.

- Characteristic cannabis withdrawal syndrome: *When you stop using cannabis, do you undergo withdrawal?*
- The same or a related substance is taken to relieve or avoid withdrawal symptoms: *Have you used cannabis or another substance to prevent withdrawal?*

b. Modifiers

i. Specifiers

- In early remission
- In sustained remission
- In a controlled environment

ii. Severity

- Mild: Use when two or three criteria are present.
- Moderate: Use when four or five criteria are present.
- Severe: Use when six or more criteria are present.

c. Alternative: If a person experiences problems associated with the use of cannabis that are not classifiable as cannabis use disorder, intoxication, withdrawal, intoxication delirium, or as a cannabis-induced psychotic disorder, anxiety disorder, or sleep disorder, consider unspecified cannabis-related disorder (see DSM-5-TR, p. 586).

7. Cannabis Intoxication

   a. Inclusion: Requires at least <u>two</u> of the following signs or symptoms.

      i. Conjunctival injection
      ii. Increased appetite: *Over the last several hours, have you been much hungrier than usual?*
      iii. Dry mouth: *Over the last several hours, have you noticed that your mouth has been dry?*
      iv. Tachycardia

   b. Inclusion: Requires clinically significant problematic behavioral or psychological changes. *Since you began this episode of cannabis use, have you observed any significant changes in your mood, judgment, ability to interact with others, or sense of time? Have you done problematic things, or thought problematic thoughts, that you would not have without cannabis?*

   c. Exclusion: If the symptoms are attributable to another medical condition or better explained by another mental disorder, including intoxication with another substance, do not make the diagnosis.

   d. Modifiers

      i. With perceptual disturbances: Use when hallucinations occur with intact reality testing or when auditory, visual, or tactile illusions occur in the absence of delirium.

8. Cannabis Withdrawal

   a. Inclusion: Requires at least <u>three</u> of the following symptoms, developing within 1 week of ceasing (or reducing) cannabis use that has been heavy and prolonged.

      i. Irritability, anger, or aggression: *Over the last week or so, have you felt more irritable or angry, or like you were ready to confront or attack someone?*
      ii. Nervousness or anxiety: *Over the last week or so, have you felt more worried or anxious than usual?*
      iii. Sleep difficulty: *Over the last week or so, have you had any disturbing dreams or found it more difficult to get to sleep and to stay asleep than usual?*

iv. Decreased appetite or weight loss: *Over the last week or so, have you been less hungry or even lost weight?*

v. Restlessness: *Over the last week or so, have you felt less able to remain at rest than usual?*

vi. Depressed mood: *Over the last week or so, have you felt more down or depressed than usual?*

vii. Somatic symptoms causing significant discomfort: *Over the last week or so, have you felt any unusual physical discomfort, such as stomach pain, tremors, sweating, fever, chills, or headaches?*

b. Exclusion: If the symptoms are attributable to another medical condition or better explained by another mental disorder, including intoxication with or withdrawal from another substance, do not make the diagnosis.

9. Phencyclidine or Other Hallucinogen Use Disorder

a. Inclusion: Requires a problematic pattern of phencyclidine or other hallucinogen use leading to clinically significant impairment or distress as manifested by at least two of the following in a 12-month period.

i. Using more phencyclidine or other hallucinogens over a longer period than intended: *When you use hallucinogens, do you find that you use more, or for a longer time, than you planned to?*

ii. Persistent desire or unsuccessful effort to reduce hallucinogen use: *Do you want to cut back or stop using hallucinogens? Have you ever tried and failed to cut back or stop using hallucinogens?*

iii. Great deal of time spent: *Do you spend a great deal of your time obtaining hallucinogens, using hallucinogens, or recovering from your hallucinogen use?*

iv. Cravings: *Do you experience strong desires or cravings to use hallucinogens?*

v. Failure to fulfill major role obligations: *Have you repeatedly failed to fulfill major obligations at work, home, or school because of your hallucinogen use?*

vi. Continued use despite awareness of interpersonal or social problems: *Do you use hallucinogens even though you suspect, or even know, that your use creates or worsens interpersonal or social problems?*

vii. Giving up activities for hallucinogens: *Are there important social, occupational, or recreational activities that*

you have given up or reduced because of your hallucinogen use?

viii. Use in hazardous situations: *Have you repeatedly
used hallucinogens in situations in which it was physically hazardous, such as driving a car or operating a machine while impaired by a hallucinogen?*

ix. Continued use despite awareness of physical or
psychological problems: *Do you use hallucinogens
even though you suspect, or even know, that they create
or worsen problems with your mind and body?*

x. Tolerance as manifested by <u>either</u> of the following.

- Markedly increased amounts: *Do you find that in
order to achieve the desired effect of hallucinogens,
you need to consume much more than you used to?*
- Markedly diminished effects: *If you use the same
amount of a hallucinogen as you used to, do you find
that it has a lot less effect on you than it used to?*

b. Modifiers

i. Specifiers

- In early remission
- In sustained remission
- In a controlled environment

ii. Severity

- Mild: Use when two or three criteria are present.
- Moderate: Use when four or five criteria are
present.
- Severe: Use when six or more criteria are present.

c. Alternatives:

i. If a person reports reexperiencing perceptual symptoms first experienced while impaired by a hallucinogen after ceasing use, consider hallucinogen
persisting perception disorder (full criteria are in
DSM-5-TR, p. 598). The symptoms must cause clinically significant distress or impairment.

ii. If a person experiences problems associated with
the use of phencyclidine or other hallucinogens that
are not classifiable as phencyclidine or other hallucinogen use disorder, intoxication, hallucinogen
persisting perception disorder, intoxication delirium, or as a phencyclidine- or other hallucinogen-

induced psychotic disorder, bipolar disorder, depressive disorder, or anxiety disorder, consider unspecified phencyclidine-related disorder or unspecified hallucinogen-related disorder (see DSM-5-TR, pp. 600–601).

10. Phencyclidine or Other Hallucinogen Intoxication

    a. Inclusion: Requires at least <u>two</u> of the following signs shortly after hallucinogen use.

Phencyclidine

      i. Vertical or horizontal nystagmus
     ii. Hypertension or tachycardia
    iii. Numbness or diminished responsiveness to pain
     iv. Ataxia
      v. Dysarthria
     vi. Muscle rigidity
    vii. Seizures or coma
   viii. Hyperacusis

Other hallucinogens

      i. Pupillary dilation
     ii. Tachycardia
    iii. Sweating: *Since taking the hallucinogen, have you noticed any change in how much you sweat?*
     iv. Palpitations: *Since taking the hallucinogen, has your heartbeat been more rapid, strong, or irregular than usual?*
      v. Blurring of vision: *Since taking the hallucinogen, has your vision been blurred?*
     vi. Tremors
    vii. Incoordination: *Since taking the hallucinogen, have you found it hard to coordinate your movements as you walk or otherwise move?*

    b. Inclusion: Requires clinically significant problematic behavioral or psychological changes. *Since you began this episode of hallucinogen use, have you observed any significant changes in your thoughts or behaviors? Have you done problematic things, or thought problematic thoughts, that you would not have without hallucinogens?*

    c. Exclusion: If the symptoms are attributable to another medical condition or better explained by another mental disorder, including intoxication with another substance, do not make the diagnosis.

11. Inhalant Use Disorder

a. Inclusion: Requires a problematic pattern of inhalant use leading to clinically significant impairment or distress as manifested by at least <u>two</u> of the following in a 12-month period.

   i. Using more inhalants over a longer period than intended: *When you inhale, do you find that you use more inhalant, or for a longer time, than you planned to?*

   ii. Persistent desire or unsuccessful effort to reduce inhalant use: *Do you want to cut back or stop inhaling? Have you ever tried and failed to cut back or stop inhaling?*

   iii. Great deal of time spent: *Do you spend a great deal of your time obtaining inhalants, using inhalants, or recovering from your inhalant use?*

   iv. Cravings: *Do you experience strong desires or cravings to use inhalants?*

   v. Failure to fulfill major role obligations: *Have you repeatedly failed to fulfill major obligations at work, home, or school because of your inhalant use?*

   vi. Continued use despite awareness of interpersonal or social problems: *Do you use inhalants even though you suspect, or even know, that your use creates or worsens interpersonal or social problems?*

   vii. Giving up activities for inhalants: *Are there important social, occupational, or recreational activities that you have given up or reduced because of your inhalant use?*

   viii. Use in hazardous situations: *Have you repeatedly used inhalants in situations in which it was physically hazardous, such as driving a car or operating a machine while high?*

   ix. Continued use despite awareness of physical or psychological problems: *Do you use inhalants even though you suspect, or even know, that it creates or worsens problems with your mind and body?*

   x. Tolerance as manifested by <u>either</u> of the following.

   - Markedly increased amounts: *Do you find that in order to get high or achieve the desired effect of using inhalants, you need to use much more than you used to?*
   - Markedly diminished effects: *If you inhale the same amount of an inhalant as you used to, do you find that it has a lot less effect on you than it used to?*

b. Modifiers

   i. Specifiers

- In early remission
- In sustained remission
- In a controlled environment

   ii. Severity

- Mild: Use when two or three criteria are present.
- Moderate: Use when four or five criteria are present.
- Severe: Use when six or more criteria are present.

c. Alternative: If a person experiences problems associated with the use of an inhalant that are not classifiable as inhalant use disorder, intoxication, intoxication delirium, or as an inhalant-induced major or mild neurocognitive disorder, psychotic disorder, depressive disorder, or anxiety disorder, consider unspecified inhalant-related disorder (see DSM-5-TR, p. 608).

12. Inhalant Intoxication

a. Inclusion: Requires at least <u>two</u> of the following signs after intended or unintended short-term, high-dose inhalant exposure.

   i. Dizziness: *Since using the inhalant, have you felt like you were reeling or about to fall?*

   ii. Nystagmus

   iii. Incoordination: *Since using the inhalant, have you found it hard to coordinate your movements as you walk or otherwise move?*

   iv. Slurred speech

   v. Unsteady gait

   vi. Lethargy: *Since using the inhalant, have you felt very sleepy or had a marked lack of energy?*

   vii. Depressed reflexes

   viii. Psychomotor retardation

   ix. Tremor

   x. Generalized muscle weakness

   xi. Blurred vision or diplopia: *Since using the inhalant, has your vision been blurred or have you been seeing double?*

   xii. Stupor or coma

   xiii. Euphoria: *Since using the inhalant, have you felt mentally or physically elated or intensely excited or happy?*

b. Inclusion: Requires clinically significant problematic behavioral or psychological changes. *Since you began this episode of inhalant use, have you observed any significant changes in your thoughts or behaviors? Have you done problematic things, or thought problematic thoughts, that you would not have without the inhalant?*

c. Exclusion: If the symptoms are attributable to another medical condition or better explained by another mental disorder, including intoxication with another substance, do not make the diagnosis.

13. Opioid Use Disorder

a. Inclusion: Requires a problematic pattern of opioid use leading to clinically significant impairment or distress as manifested by at least <u>two</u> of the following in a 12-month period.

   i. Using more opioids over a longer period than intended: *When you use opioids, do you find that you use more, or for a longer time, than you planned to?*

   ii. Persistent desire or unsuccessful effort to reduce opioid use: *Do you want to cut back or stop using opioids? Have you ever tried and failed to cut back or stop your opioid use?*

   iii. Great deal of time spent: *Do you spend a great deal of your time obtaining opioids, using opioids, or recovering from your opioid use?*

   iv. Cravings: *Do you experience strong desires or cravings to use opioids?*

   v. Failure to fulfill major role obligations: *Have you repeatedly failed to fulfill major obligations at work, home, or school because of your opioid use?*

   vi. Continued use despite awareness of interpersonal or social problems: *Do you continue to use opioids even though you suspect, or even know, that your use creates or worsens interpersonal or social problems?*

   vii. Giving up activities for opioids: *Are there important social, occupational, or recreational activities that you have given up or reduced because of your opioid use?*

   viii. Use in hazardous situations: *Have you repeatedly used opioids in situations in which it was physically hazardous, such as driving a car or operating a machine while intoxicated?*

   ix. Continued use despite awareness of physical or psychological problems: *Do you use opioids even though you suspect, or even know, that it creates or worsens problems with your mind and body?*

 x. Tolerance as manifested by <u>either</u> of the following.

  • Markedly increased amounts: *Do you find that in order to get high or achieve the desired effect of using opioids, you need to consume much more than you used to?*

  • Markedly diminished effects (excluding opioid medications taken under medical supervision): *If you use the same amount of an opioid as you used to, do you find that it has a lot less effect on you than it used to?*

 xi. Withdrawal as manifested by <u>either</u> of the following.

  • Characteristic opioid withdrawal syndrome: *When you stop using opioids, do you undergo withdrawal?*

  • The same or a closely related substance is taken to relieve or avoid withdrawal symptoms: *Have you ever taken opioids or another substance to prevent opioid withdrawal?*

b. Modifiers

 i. Specifiers

  • In early remission
  • In sustained remission
  • On maintenance therapy
  • In a controlled environment

 ii. Severity

  • Mild: Use when two or three criteria are present.
  • Moderate: Use when four or five criteria are present.
  • Severe: Use when six or more criteria are present.

c. Alternative: If a person experiences problems associated with the use of opioids that are not classifiable as opioid use disorder, intoxication, withdrawal, intoxication delirium, withdrawal delirium, or a an opioid-induced psychotic disorder, bipolar disorder, depressive disorder, anxiety disorder, sexual dysfunction, or sleep disorder, consider unspecified opioid-related disorder (see DSM-5-TR, p. 619).

14. Opioid Intoxication

   a. Inclusion: Requires pupillary constriction shortly after opioid use and at least <u>one</u> of the following signs.

      i. Drowsiness or coma
      ii. Slurred speech
      iii. Impairment in attention or memory

   b. Inclusion: Requires clinically significant problematic behavioral or psychological changes. *Since you began this episode of opioid use, have you observed any significant changes in your thoughts or behaviors? Have you done problematic things, or thought problematic thoughts, that you would not have without the opioid?*

   c. Exclusion: If the symptoms are attributable to another medical condition or better explained by another mental disorder, including intoxication with another substance, do not make the diagnosis.

   d. Modifiers

      i. With perceptual disturbances: Use when hallucinations occur with intact reality testing or when auditory, visual, or tactile illusions occur in the absence of delirium.

15. Opioid Withdrawal

   a. Inclusion: Requires at least <u>three</u> of the following symptoms, developing within minutes to several days of ceasing (or reducing) opioid use that has been heavy and prolonged OR following the administration of an opioid antagonist after a period of opioid use.

      i. Dysphoric mood: *Over the last couple of days, have you been feeling more down or depressed than usual?*

      ii. Nausea or vomiting: *Over the last couple of days, have you felt sick to your stomach, felt nauseated, or even vomited?*

      iii. Muscle aches: *Over the last couple of days, have you experienced muscle aches or pains?*

      iv. Lacrimation or rhinorrhea: *Over the last couple of days, have you noticed that you have been shedding tears when you did not feel like crying? Have you noticed that your nose has been running, or discharging clear fluid, more than usual?*

v. Pupillary dilation, piloerection, or sweating

vi. Diarrhea: *Over the last couple of days, have you experienced more frequent or more liquid stools than usual?*

vii. Yawning: *Over the last couple of days, have you been yawning much more than usual?*

viii. Fever

ix. Insomnia: *Over the last couple of days, have you found it more difficult than usual to get to sleep and to stay asleep?*

b. Exclusion: If the symptoms are attributable to another medical condition or better explained by another mental disorder, including intoxication with or withdrawal from another substance, do not make the diagnosis.

16. Sedative, Hypnotic, or Anxiolytic Use Disorder

a. Inclusion: Requires a problematic pattern of sedative, hypnotic, or anxiolytic use leading to clinically significant impairment or distress as manifested by at least <u>two</u> of the following in a 12-month period.

i. Using more sedatives, hypnotics, or anxiolytics over a longer period than intended: *When you use sedatives, hypnotics, or anxiolytics, do you find that you use more, and for a longer time, than you planned to?*

ii. Persistent desire or unsuccessful effort to reduce sedative, hypnotic, or anxiolytic use: *Do you want to cut back or stop using sedatives, hypnotics, or anxiolytics? Have you ever tried and failed to cut back or stop using sedatives, hypnotics, or anxiolytics?*

iii. Great deal of time spent: *Do you spend a great deal of your time obtaining and using sedatives, hypnotics, or anxiolytics or recovering from your sedative, hypnotic, or anxiolytic use?*

iv. Cravings: *Do you experience strong desires or cravings to use sedatives, hypnotics, or anxiolytics?*

v. Failure to fulfill major role obligations: *Have you repeatedly failed to fulfill major obligations at work, home, or school because of your sedative, hypnotic, or anxiolytic use?*

vi. Continued use despite awareness of interpersonal or social problems: *Do you use a sedative, hypnotic, or anxiolytic even though you suspect, or even know, that it creates or worsens interpersonal or social problems?*

vii. Giving up activities for sedatives, hypnotics, or anxiolytics: *Are there important social, occupational, or recreational activities that you have given up or reduced because of your sedative, hypnotic, or anxiolytic use?*

viii. Use in hazardous situations: *Have you repeatedly used a sedative, hypnotic, or anxiolytic in situations in which it was physically hazardous, such as driving a car or operating a machine while impaired by sedative use?*

ix. Continued use despite awareness of physical or psychological problems: *Do you use sedatives, hypnotics, or anxiolytics even though you suspect, or even know, that your use creates or worsens problems with your mind and body?*

x. Tolerance as manifested by <u>either</u> of the following.

- Markedly increased amounts: *Do you find that in order to get intoxicated or achieve the desired effect of using sedatives, hypnotics, or anxiolytics, you need to consume much more than you used to?*
- Markedly diminished effects: *If you use the same amount of a sedative, hypnotic, or anxiolytic as you used to, do you find that it has a lot less effect on you than it used to?*

xi. Withdrawal as manifested by <u>either</u> of the following.

- Characteristic sedative, hypnotic, or anxiolytic withdrawal syndrome: *When you stop using sedatives, hypnotics, or anxiolytics, do you undergo withdrawal?*
- The same or a closely related substance is taken to relieve or avoid withdrawal symptoms: *Have you ever taken sedatives, hypnotics, anxiolytics, or another substance to prevent withdrawal?*

b. Modifiers

i. Specifiers

- In early remission
- In sustained remission
- In a controlled environment

ii. Severity

- Mild: Use when two or three criteria are present.
- Moderate: Use when four or five criteria are present.
- Severe: Use when six or more criteria are present.

c. Alternative: If a person experiences problems associated with the use of a sedative, hypnotic, or anxiolytic that are not classifiable as sedative, hypnotic, or anxiolytic use disorder, intoxication, withdrawal, intoxication delirium, withdrawal delirium, or as a sedative-, hypnotic-, or anxiolytic-induced major or mild neurocognitive disorder, psychotic disorder, bipolar disorder, depressive disorder, anxiety disorder, sexual dysfunction, or sleep disorder, consider unspecified sedative-, hypnotic-, or anxiolytic-related disorder (see DSM-5-TR, p. 632).

17. Sedative, Hypnotic, or Anxiolytic Intoxication

   a. Inclusion: Requires <u>one</u> of the following signs shortly after sedative, hypnotic, or anxiolytic use.

      i. Slurred speech
      ii. Incoordination
      iii. Unsteady gait
      iv. Nystagmus
      v. Impairment in cognition (i.e., attention or memory)
      vi. Stupor or coma

   b. Inclusion: Requires clinically significant problematic behavioral or psychological changes. *Since you began this episode of sedative, hypnotic, or anxiolytic use, have you observed any significant changes in your thoughts or behaviors? Have you done problematic things, or thought problematic thoughts, that you would not have without the sedative, hypnotic, or anxiolytic?*

   c. Exclusion: If the symptoms are attributable to another medical condition or better explained by another mental disorder, including intoxication with another substance, do not make the diagnosis.

18. Sedative, Hypnotic, or Anxiolytic Withdrawal

   a. Inclusion: Requires at least <u>two</u> of the following symptoms, developing within several hours to a few days after ceasing (or reducing) sedative, hypnotic, or anxiolytic use that has been heavy and prolonged.

      i. Autonomic hyperactivity
      ii. Hand tremor
      iii. Insomnia: *Over the last couple of days, have you found it more difficult than usual to get to sleep or to stay asleep?*

    iv. Nausea or vomiting: *Over the last couple of days, have you felt sick to your stomach, felt nauseated, or even vomited?*

    v. Transient visual, tactile, or auditory hallucinations or illusions: *Over the last couple of days, have you had any experiences where you worried that your mind was playing tricks on you, like seeing, hearing, or feeling things that other people could not?*

    vi. Psychomotor agitation

    vii. Anxiety: *Over the last couple of days, have you felt more worried or anxious than usual?*

    viii. Grand mal seizures

b. Exclusion: If the symptoms are attributable to another medical condition or better explained by another mental disorder, including intoxication with or withdrawal from another substance, do not make the diagnosis.

c. Modifiers

    i. Specifiers

      • With perceptual disturbances: Use when hallucinations occur with intact reality testing or when auditory, visual, or tactile illusions occur in the absence of delirium.

d. Alternative: If a person experiences problems associated with the use of a sedative, hypnotic, or anxiolytic that are not classifiable as a sedative-, hypnotic-, or anxiolytic-related disorder, consider unspecified sedative-, hypnotic-, or anxiolytic-related disorder (see DSM-5-TR, p. 632).

19. Stimulant Use Disorder

a. Inclusion: Requires a problematic pattern of stimulant use leading to clinically significant impairment or distress as manifested by at least <u>two</u> of the following in a 12-month period.

    i. Using more stimulants over a longer period than intended: *When you use stimulants, do you find that you use more, or for a longer time, than you planned to?*

    ii. Persistent desire or unsuccessful effort to reduce stimulant use: *Do you want to cut back or stop using stimulants? Have you ever tried and failed to cut back or stop using stimulants?*

iii. Great deal of time spent: *Do you spend a great deal of your time obtaining stimulants, using stimulants, or recovering from your stimulant use?*

iv. Cravings: *Do you experience strong desires or cravings to use stimulants?*

v. Failure to fulfill major role obligations: *Have you repeatedly failed to fulfill major obligations at work, home, or school because of your stimulant use?*

vi. Continued use despite awareness of interpersonal or social problems: *Do you use stimulants even though you suspect, or even know, that your use creates or worsens interpersonal or social problems?*

vii. Giving up activities for stimulants: *Are there important social, occupational, or recreational activities that you have given up or reduced because of your stimulant use?*

viii. Use in hazardous situations: *Have you repeatedly used stimulants in situations in which it was physically hazardous, such as driving a car or operating a machine while intoxicated?*

ix. Continued use despite awareness of physical or psychological problems: *Do you use stimulants even though you suspect, or even know, that it creates or worsens problems with your mind and body?*

x. Tolerance as manifested by either of the following. **Note:** This criterion is not met if taking stimulants as prescribed under medical supervision.

• Markedly increased amounts: *Do you find that in order to get intoxicated or achieve the desired effect of using stimulants, you need to consume much more than you used to?*

• Markedly diminished effects: *If you use the same amount of a stimulant as you used to, do you find that it has a lot less effect on you than it used to?*

xi. Withdrawal as manifested by either of the following. **Note:** This criterion is not met if taking stimulants as prescribed under medical supervision.

• Characteristic stimulant withdrawal syndrome: *When you stop using stimulants, do you undergo withdrawal?*

• The same or a closely related substance is taken to relieve or avoid withdrawal symptoms: *Have you ever taken stimulants or another substance to prevent withdrawal?*

b. Modifiers

    i. Specify stimulant

- Amphetamine-type substance
- Cocaine
- Other or unspecified stimulant

    ii. Specifiers

- In early remission
- In sustained remission
- In a controlled environment

    iii. Severity

- Mild: Use when two or three criteria are present.
- Moderate: Use when four or five criteria are present.
- Severe: Use when six or more criteria are present.

c. Alternative: If a person experiences problems associated with the use of stimulants that are not classifiable as stimulant use disorder, intoxication, withdrawal, intoxication delirium, or as a stimulant-induced psychotic disorder, bipolar disorder, depressive disorder, anxiety disorder, sexual dysfunction, or sleep disorder, consider unspecified stimulant-related disorder (see DSM-5-TR, p. 644).

20. Stimulant Intoxication

a. Inclusion: Requires at least <u>two</u> of the following signs shortly after stimulant use.

    i. Tachycardia or bradycardia
    ii. Pupillary dilation
    iii. Elevated or lowered blood pressure
    iv. Perspiration or chills: *Over the last couple of hours, have you experienced chills or been sweating more than usual?*
    v. Nausea or vomiting: *Over the last couple of hours, have you felt sick to your stomach, felt nauseated, or even vomited?*
    vi. Evidence of weight loss
    vii. Psychomotor agitation
    viii. Muscular weakness, respiratory depression, chest pain, or cardiac arrhythmias
    ix. Confusion, seizures, dyskinesias, dystonias, or coma

b. Inclusion: Requires clinically significant problematic behavioral or psychological changes. *Since you began this episode of stimulant use, have you observed any significant changes in your thoughts or behaviors? Have you done problematic things, or thought problematic thoughts, that you would not have without the stimulant?*

c. Exclusion: If the symptoms are attributable to another medical condition or better explained by another mental disorder, including intoxication with another substance, do not make the diagnosis.

d. Modifiers

  i. Specifiers

   • With perceptual disturbances: Use when hallucinations occur with intact reality testing or when auditory, visual, or tactile illusions occur in the absence of delirium.
   • Amphetamine-type substance or cocaine

21. Stimulant Withdrawal

a. Inclusion: Requires the following symptom, developing within hours to days of ceasing (or reducing) stimulant use that has been heavy and prolonged.

  i. Dysphoric mood: *Over the last few hours or days, have you felt much more down or depressed than usual?*

b. Inclusion: Also requires at least <u>two</u> of the following symptoms.

  i. Fatigue: *Over the last few hours or days, have you felt extremely sleepy or tired?*

  ii. Vivid, unpleasant dreams: *Over the last few hours or days, have you experienced unusually vivid, unpleasant dreams?*

  iii. Insomnia or hypersomnia: *Over the last few hours or days, have you found it more difficult than usual to get to sleep and to stay asleep? Alternatively, have you found that you have been sleeping much more than usual?*

  iv. Increased appetite: *Over the last few hours or days, have you desired food much more than usual?*

  v. Psychomotor retardation or agitation

c. Exclusion: If the symptoms are attributable to another medical condition or better explained by another mental disorder, including intoxication with or withdrawal from another substance, do not make the diagnosis.

d. Modifiers

  i. Amphetamine-type substance or cocaine

e. Alternative: If a person experiences problems associated with the use of a stimulant that are not classifiable as a stimulant-related disorder, consider unspecified stimulant-related disorder (see DSM-5-TR, p. 644).

22. Tobacco Use Disorder

a. Inclusion: Requires a problematic pattern of tobacco use leading to clinically significant impairment or distress as manifested by at least <u>two</u> of the following in a 12-month period.

   i. Using more tobacco over a longer period than intended: *When you use tobacco, do you find that you use more, or for a longer time, than you planned to?*

   ii. Persistent desire or unsuccessful effort to reduce tobacco use: *Do you want to cut back or stop using tobacco? Have you ever tried and failed to cut back or stop using tobacco?*

   iii. Great deal of time spent: *Do you spend a great deal of your time obtaining tobacco, using tobacco, or recovering from your tobacco use?*

   iv. Cravings: *Do you experience strong desires or cravings to use tobacco?*

   v. Failure to fulfill major role obligations: *Have you repeatedly failed to fulfill major obligations at work, home, or school because of your tobacco use?*

   vi. Continued use despite awareness of interpersonal or social problems: *Do you use tobacco even though you suspect, or even know, that your use creates or worsens interpersonal or social problems?*

   vii. Giving up activities for tobacco: *Are there important social, occupational, or recreational activities that you have given up or reduced because of your tobacco use?*

   viii. Use in hazardous situations: *Have you repeatedly used tobacco in situations in which it was physically hazardous, like smoking in bed?*

   ix. Continued use despite awareness of physical or psychological problems: *Do you use tobacco even though you suspect, or even know, that it creates or worsens problems with your mind and body?*

   x. Tolerance as manifested by <u>either</u> of the following.

     • Markedly increased amounts: *Do you find that in order to get the desired effect of tobacco, you need to use much more than you used to?*

The DSM-5-TR Diagnostic Interview   **157**

- Markedly diminished effects: *If you use the same amount of tobacco as you used to, do you find that it has a lot less effect on you than it used to?*

   xi. Withdrawal as manifested by <u>either</u> of the following.

- Characteristic tobacco withdrawal syndrome: *When you stop using tobacco, do you undergo withdrawal?*
- The same substance is taken to relieve or avoid withdrawal symptoms: *Have you ever used tobacco to avoid or relieve symptoms of tobacco withdrawal?*

  b. Modifiers

     i. Specifiers

- In early remission
- In sustained remission
- On maintenance therapy
- In a controlled environment

    ii. Severity

- Mild: Use when two or three criteria are present.
- Moderate: Use when four or five criteria are present.
- Severe: Use when six or more criteria are present.

23. Tobacco Withdrawal

  a. Inclusion: Requires at least <u>four</u> of the following symptoms, developing within 24 hours of ceasing (or reducing) tobacco use that has been daily for at least several weeks.

     i. Irritability, frustration, or anger: *Over the last 24 hours, have you felt more irritable, frustrated, or angry than usual?*

    ii. Anxiety: *Over the last 24 hours, have you felt more worried or anxious than usual?*

   iii. Difficulty concentrating: *Over the last 24 hours, have you had difficulty staying focused on a task or activity?*

   iv. Increased appetite: *Over the last 24 hours, have you desired food more than usual?*

    v. Restlessness: *Over the last 24 hours, have you felt less able to remain at rest than usual?*

   vi. Depressed mood: *Over the last 24 hours, have you been feeling more down or depressed than usual?*

vii. Insomnia: *Over the last 24 hours, have you found it more difficult than usual to get to sleep or to stay asleep?*

b. Exclusion: If the symptoms are attributable to another medical condition or better explained by another mental disorder, including intoxication with or withdrawal from another substance, do not make the diagnosis.

c. Alternative: If a person experiences problems associated with the use of tobacco that are not classifiable as a tobacco-related disorder, consider unspecified tobacco-related disorder (see DSM-5-TR, p. 651).

24. Other (or Unknown) Substance Use Disorder

a. Inclusion: Requires a problematic pattern of use of an intoxicating substance not able to be classified within the other substance categories above, leading to clinically significant impairment or distress as manifested by at least <u>two</u> of the following in a 12-month period.

i. Taking more of the substance over a longer period than intended: *When you use the substance, do you find that you use it more often, or for a longer time, than you planned to?*

ii. Persistent desire or unsuccessful effort to reduce substance use: *Do you want to cut back or stop using the substance? Have you ever tried and failed to cut back or stop using the substance?*

iii. Great deal of time spent: *Do you spend a great deal of your time obtaining or using the substance or recovering from your substance use?*

iv. Cravings: *Do you experience strong desires or cravings to use the substance?*

v. Failure to fulfill major role obligations: *Have you repeatedly failed to fulfill major obligations at work, home, or school because of your substance use?*

vi. Continued use despite awareness of interpersonal or social problems: *Do you use the substance even though you suspect, or even know, that it creates or worsens interpersonal or social problems?*

vii. Giving up activities for the substance: *Are there important social, occupational, or recreational activities that you have given up or reduced because of your substance use?*

viii. Use in hazardous situations: *Have you repeatedly used the substance in situations in which it was physi-*

cally hazardous, such as driving a car or operating a machine while intoxicated?

ix. Continued use despite awareness of physical or psychological problems: *Do you use the substance even though you suspect, or even know, that it creates or worsens problems with your mind and body?*

x. Tolerance as manifested by <u>either</u> of the following.

- Markedly increased amounts: *Do you find that in order to get intoxicated or achieve the desired effect of substance use, you need to consume much more of the substance than you used to?*
- Markedly diminished effects: *If you use the same amount of the substance as you used to, do you find that it has a lot less effect on you than it used to?*

xi. Withdrawal as manifested by <u>either</u> of the following.

- Characteristic withdrawal syndrome for the substance: *When you stop using the substance, do you undergo withdrawal?*
- The same or a closely related substance is taken to relieve or avoid withdrawal symptoms: *Have you ever taken the substance or another substance to prevent withdrawal?*

b. Modifiers

i. Specifiers

- In early remission
- In sustained remission
- In a controlled environment

ii. Severity

- Mild: Use when two or three symptoms are present.
- Moderate: Use when four or five symptoms are present.
- Severe: Use when six or more symptoms are present.

c. Alternatives

i. If a person experiences problems associated with use of the substance that are not classifiable as other (or unknown) substance use disorder, substance intoxication, or withdrawal, consider unspecified other (or unknown) substance–related disorder (see DSM-5-TR, pp. 660–661).

25. Other (or Unknown) Substance Intoxication

   a. Inclusion: Development of a reversible substance-specific syndrome attributable to recent ingestion of (or exposure to) a substance that is not listed elsewhere or is unknown.

   b. Inclusion: Requires clinically significant problematic behavioral or psychological changes. *Since you began this episode of substance use, have you observed any significant changes in your behavior, mood, or judgment? Have you done problematic things, or thought problematic thoughts, that you would not have if you were not using the substance?*

   c. Exclusion: If the symptoms are attributable to another medical condition or are better explained by another mental disorder, including intoxication with another substance, do not make the diagnosis.

26. Other (or Unknown) Substance Withdrawal

   a. Inclusion: Development of a substance-specific syndrome shortly after the cessation of (or reduction in) use of the substance that has been heavy and prolonged.

   b. Inclusion: Requires clinically significant distress or impairment in social, occupational, or other important areas of functioning.

   c. Exclusion: If the symptoms are attributable to another medical condition or are better explained by another mental disorder, including withdrawal from another substance, do not make the diagnosis.

27. Gambling Disorder

   a. Inclusion: Requires persistent, recurrent problematic gaming that leads to clinically significant impairment or distress, lasting at least 12 months, as indicated by at least <u>four</u> of the following symptoms.

      i. Escalates spending on gambling: *Do you find that it takes increasing amounts of money to get the excitement you want from gambling?*

      ii. Is irritable when quitting: *When you try to reduce or quit gambling, are you irritable or restless?*

      iii. Is unable to quit: *Have you unsuccessfully tried to reduce or quit gambling on several occasions?*

iv. Is preoccupied: *Are you preoccupied with gambling?*

v. Gambles when distressed: *When you are feeling anxious, down, or helpless, do you gamble?*

vi. Chases losses: *After you lose money, do you return another day to try to get even?*

vii. Lies: *Do you lie to conceal how much you gamble?*

viii. Loses relationships: *Have you lost a relationship, job, or opportunity because of your gambling?*

ix. Borrows money: *Do you have to rely on other people for money to cover desperate financial situations caused by gambling?*

b. Exclusion: If the gambling behavior is better accounted for by a manic episode, do not make the diagnosis.

c. Modifiers

i. Course

- Episodic: Meeting diagnostic criteria at more than one time point, with symptoms subsiding between periods of gambling disorder for at least several months
- Persistent: Experiencing continuous symptoms to meet diagnostic criteria for multiple years
- In early remission
- In sustained remission

ii. Severity

- Mild: Use when four or five criteria are met.
- Moderate: Use when six or seven criteria are met.
- Severe: Use when eight or nine criteria are met.

Neurocognitive Disorders

DSM-5-TR pp. 667–732

Screening questions: Use orientation and Mini-Cog questions. *I am going to say three words that I want you to repeat back to me now and try to remember. The words are: river, nation, finger. Please say them for me now.* Then say: *Now I would like you to draw a clock for me. First, put in all of the numbers where they go.* When the clock-drawing task is completed, say: *Now, set the hands to 10 past 11.* Finally, ask: *What were the three words I asked you to remember?*

- If a person is disoriented, proceed to delirium criteria.
- If a person is oriented but experiencing cognitive difficulties, ask: *Are you able to live as independently as you used to? For example, can you cook like you used to, and keep track of your medications and your finances like you used to?*
- If a person answers yes, proceed to mild neurocognitive disorder criteria.
- If a person, or his caregiver, answers no, proceed to major neurocognitive disorder criteria.

1. Delirium

   a. Inclusion: Requires the presence of all <u>three</u> of the following disturbances, which are usually assessed by means of the examination and validated instruments (e.g., Inouye et al. 1990), rather than through diagnostic questions.

      i. Disturbance in attention as manifested by reduced ability to direct, focus, sustain, and shift attention and a reduction in environmental awareness

      ii. Disturbance that represents an acute change from baseline and that developed over a short period of time (hours to days), and with severity that tends to fluctuate during the day

      iii. Change in cognition, such as memory deficit, disorientation, language disturbance, visuospatial ability, or perception

   b. Exclusions

      i. If the change in cognition is better accounted for by a preexisting, established, or evolving neurocognitive disorder, do not make the diagnosis.

      ii. If the disturbance in cognition occurs in the context of a severely reduced level of arousal, such as coma, do not make the diagnosis.

      iii. If the disturbance in cognition is a physiological consequence of another medical condition, substance intoxication or withdrawal, or exposure to a toxin, or is due to multiple etiologies, do not make the diagnosis.

   c. Modifiers

      i. Subtypes

         - Substance intoxication delirium: Use when delirium is the predominating experience of a person's intoxication and inclusion criteria (i) and (iii) above predominate.

- Substance withdrawal delirium: Use when delirium is the predominating experience of a person's withdrawal and inclusion criteria (i) and (iii) above predominate.
- Medication-induced delirium: Use when inclusion criteria (ii) and (iii) arise as a side effect of a medication taken as prescribed.
- Delirium due to another medical condition
- Delirium due to multiple etiologies

  ii. Specifiers

- Course

  - Acute: Lasting a few hours or days
  - Persistent: Lasting weeks or months

- Descriptive features

  - Hyperactive
  - Hypoactive
  - Mixed level of activity

  d. Alternative: If you are unable to determine why a person is experiencing delirium, or if his delirium is subsyndromal, consider unspecified delirium (see DSM-5-TR, p. 678). If you wish to communicate the specific reason a person's symptoms do not meet full criteria for delirium, consider other specified delirium (see DSM-5-TR, p. 678). An example is subsyndromal delirium.

2. Major Neurocognitive Disorder

  a. Inclusion: Requires evidence of significant cognitive decline from a previous level of performance in one or more cognitive domains based on <u>both</u> of the following, which are usually assessed using the examination rather than through diagnostic questions.

    i. A person's self-concern, or the concern of a knowledgeable informant or the clinician, that a significant cognitive decline has occurred
    ii. A substantial impairment in cognitive performance, preferably documented by standardized neuropsychological testing or, in its absence, another quantified clinical assessment

b. Inclusion: Also, the cognitive deficits interfere with independence in everyday activities.

c. Exclusion: If the cognitive impairments occur exclusively while the patient is delirious or are primarily the result of another mental disorder, do not make the diagnosis.

d. Modifiers

   i. Subtypes: Specify whether due to:

   - Alzheimer's disease: Characteristically associated with an insidious onset and gradual progression, in which memory impairment is an early and prominent feature. Requires exclusion of other known neurocognitive disorders. (Full criteria are in DSM-5-TR, pp. 690–691.)
   - Frontotemporal degeneration: Requires evidence for the characteristic impairments associated with behavioral or language variants. The behavioral variant can include prominent decline in social cognition and/or executive abilities; disinhibition; apathy or inertia; loss of sympathy or empathy; perseverative, stereotyped, or compulsive/ritualistic behavior; and hyperorality and dietary changes. The language variant includes prominent decline in language ability, in the form of speech production, word finding, object naming, grammar, or word comprehension. In both variants, learning, memory, and perceptual motor function are relatively spared. Requires the exclusion of another neurocognitive disorder. (Full criteria are in DSM-5-TR, pp. 695–696.)
   - Lewy body disease: Requires evidence of fluctuating cognition with pronounced variations in attention and alertness, recurrent visual hallucinations that are typically well formed and detailed, and spontaneous features of parkinsonism with onset of motor symptoms at least 1 year later than the cognitive impairment. Requires the exclusion of another neurocognitive disorder. (Full criteria are in DSM-5-TR, pp. 699–700.)
   - Vascular disease: Requires evidence of cerebrovascular disease and exclusion of other known neurocognitive disorders. Deficits in the speed

of information processing, complex attention, or frontal-executive functioning are characteristic. Onset is temporally related to one or more cerebrovascular events. (Full criteria are in DSM-5-TR, pp. 702–703.)

- Traumatic brain injury: Requires an impact to the head or other rapid displacement of the brain within the skull that results in <u>one</u> or more of the following: loss of consciousness, posttraumatic amnesia, disorientation and confusion, or neurological signs (e.g., visual field cuts, hemiparesis, hemisensory loss, cortical blindness, aphasia, apraxia, weakness, loss of balance). The cognitive deficits present immediately following the injury or after recovery of consciousness and persist past the acute post-injury period (i.e., for at least 1 week). (Full criteria are in DSM-5-TR, pp. 706–707.)

- Substance/medication use: Requires presumptive evidence of an etiological relationship between past or present substance use and cognitive deficits. A person must have used a substance or medication for a duration and extent capable of producing the neurocognitive impairment. Requires the exclusion of another medical condition or mental disorder or current intoxication or withdrawal. (Full criteria are in DSM-5-TR, pp. 712–713.)

- HIV infection: Requires documented infection with HIV. Symptoms cannot be better explained by secondary brain diseases like progressive multifocal leukoencephalopathy or cryptococcal meningitis. Requires the exclusion of another neurocognitive disorder. (Full criteria are in DSM-5-TR, pp. 717–718.)

- Prion disease: Requires evidence that the neurocognitive disorder is due to a prion disease. Requires the presence of motor features of prion disease or biomarker evidence. Requires the exclusion of cognitive deficits due to delirium or another mental disorder. (Full criteria are in DSM-5-TR, p. 721.)

- Parkinson's disease: Requires the established presence of Parkinson's disease and the insidious onset and gradual progression of impairing cognitive deficits. (Full criteria are in DSM-5-TR, pp. 723–724.)
- Huntington's disease: Requires the presence of clinically established Huntington's disease or evidence of risk for the disease based on family history or genetic testing, and the insidious onset and gradual progression of impairing cognitive deficits. (Full criteria are in DSM-5-TR, pp. 726–727.)
- Another medical condition: Requires evidence that the neurocognitive disorder is the pathophysiological consequence of another medical condition. Requires the exclusion of cognitive deficits due to delirium or another mental disorder. (Full criteria are in DSM-5-TR, pp. 729–730.)
- Multiple etiologies: Requires evidence from the history, physical examination, or laboratory findings that the neurocognitive disorder is the pathophysiological consequence of more than one etiological process, excluding substances. Requires the exclusion of cognitive deficits due to delirium or another mental disorder. (Full criteria are in DSM-5-TR, p. 731.)
- Unspecified: Can be used in the event of a subthreshold syndrome, an atypical presentation, an uncertain etiology, or a specific syndrome not listed in DSM-5-TR. (See DSM-5-TR, p. 732.)

ii. Specifiers

- Without behavioral disturbance
- With behavioral disturbance

iii. Severity

- Mild: Use when some difficulties with instrumental activities of daily living are present.
- Moderate: Use when difficulties with basic activities of daily living are present.
- Severe: Use when a person is fully dependent on other people.

3. Mild Neurocognitive Disorder

   a. Inclusion: Requires evidence of significant cognitive decline from a previous level of performance in one or more cognitive domains based on <u>both</u> of the following, which are usually assessed using the examination rather than through diagnostic questions.

      i. A person's self-concern, or the concern of a knowledgeable informant or the clinician, that a significant cognitive decline has occurred
      ii. A substantial impairment in cognitive performance, preferably documented by standardized neuropsychological testing or, in its absence, another quantified clinical assessment

   b. Inclusion: Also, the cognitive deficits do not interfere with capacity for independence in everyday activities (but greater effort, compensatory strategies, or accommodation may be required).

   c. Exclusion: If the cognitive impairments occur exclusively while the patient is delirious or are primarily the result of another mental disorder, do not make the diagnosis.

   d. Modifiers

      i. Subtypes (see full descriptions in major neurocognitive disorder above): Specify whether due to:
          • Alzheimer's disease
          • Frontotemporal degeneration
          • Lewy body disease
          • Vascular disease
          • Traumatic brain injury
          • Substance/medication use
          • HIV infection
          • Prion disease
          • Parkinson's disease
          • Huntington's disease
          • Another medical condition
          • Multiple etiologies
          • Unspecified

      ii. Specifiers
          • Without behavioral disturbance
          • With behavioral disturbance

Personality Disorders

DSM-5-TR pp. 733–778

Screening questions: *When anyone reflects on their life, they can identify patterns—characteristic thoughts, moods, and actions—that began when they were a young person and have subsequently occurred in many personal and social situations. Thinking about your own life, can you identify patterns that have caused you significant problems with your friends or family, at work, or in another setting?*

   If yes, ask: *When you think about these characteristic patterns of behavior that began when you were a young person, can you recognize enduring patterns in the way you perceive yourself and other people, the ways you respond emotionally to exciting or difficult circumstances, the ways you interact with other people, or your ability to control your impulses and urges?*

   If yes, ask: *When you look over your life, can you see that one or more of the following ways of being has been relatively stable over time?*

- *Distrusting other people and suspecting them of wishing evil upon you*
  - If distrust and suspiciousness of others predominate, proceed to paranoid personality disorder criteria.
- *Feeling disconnected from close relationships and preferring not to express much emotion*
  - If detachment and restricted range of emotions predominate, proceed to schizoid personality disorder criteria.
- *Feeling uncomfortable in close relationships and preferring activities that many other people consider unusual or eccentric*
  - If discomfort in close relationships and eccentric behavior predominate, proceed to schizotypal personality disorder criteria.
- *Disregarding the rights of other people without concern for how it affects them*
  - If disregard for the rights of other people predominates, proceed to antisocial personality disorder criteria.
- *Experiencing yourself, your mood, and your relationships as constantly changing*

- If instability in relationships, self-image, and affects predominates, proceed to borderline personality disorder criteria.

- *Being more emotional and desiring more attention than other people*

    - If excessive emotionality and attention-seeking predominate, proceed to histrionic personality disorder criteria.

- *Sensing that you are much more accomplished or deserving than other people*

    - If grandiosity and need for admiration predominate, proceed to narcissistic personality disorder criteria.

- *Avoiding other people because you feel inferior or fear they will criticize or reject you*

    - If social inhibition and feelings of inadequacy predominate, proceed to avoidant personality disorder criteria.

- *Wanting so much for someone to take care of you that you become submissive or clingy and repeatedly fear they will separate from you*

    - If a need to be taken care of predominates, proceed to dependent personality disorder criteria.

- *Focusing on getting things rightly ordered, perfect, or in control*

    - If preoccupation with orderliness, perfectionism, and control predominates, proceed to obsessive-compulsive personality disorder criteria.

1. Paranoid Personality Disorder

    a. Inclusion: Requires a pervasive pattern of distrust and suspiciousness of others such that their motives are interpreted as malevolent, as indicated by at least <u>four</u> of the following manifestations.

        i. Suspects exploitation or harm: *Do you frequently suspect that other people are exploiting, harming, or deceiving you, even when you have limited evidence for these suspicions?*

        ii. Preoccupied with doubts: *Do you find that thinking about whether or not the people in your life are loyal or trustworthy dominates your thoughts?*

        iii. Reluctant to confide: *Are you often reluctant to tell someone about a personal or private matter because you fear they will use the information to harm you?*

    iv. Reads hidden meanings: *Do often feel that when people talk about you they are demeaning or threatening you?*

    v. Persistently bears grudges: *When someone insults, injures, or slights you, do you bear a grudge and find it very hard to forgive?*

    vi. Perceives character attacks: *Do you find that other people often say or do things to attack your character or reputation? Do you counterattack or react angrily to people?*

    vii. Suspects infidelity: *When you are involved in a relationship, do you repeatedly suspect your partner of being unfaithful to you, without having any evidence?*

  b. Exclusion: If the disturbance occurs exclusively in the course of a psychotic disorder, or a bipolar or depressive disorder with psychotic features, or is a physiological effect of another medical condition, do not make the diagnosis.

2. Schizoid Personality Disorder

  a. Inclusion: Requires a pervasive pattern of detachment from social relationships and a restricted range of expression of emotions in interpersonal settings, as indicated by at least <u>four</u> of the following manifestations.

    i. Neither desires nor enjoys close relationships: *Do you find that you neither desire to be nor enjoy being close to other people, including your family?*

    ii. Chooses solitary activities: *When you have a choice, do you almost always choose activities that you can do without other people?*

    iii. Little interest in sexual experiences with others: *Would it be okay with you if you lived the rest of your life without romantic or sexual experiences with other people?*

    iv. Takes pleasure in few activities: *Do you find that very few activities bring you pleasure or enjoyment?*

    v. Lacks close friends and confidants: *Other than your immediate family, do you find that you do not have close friends or people with whom you share personal matters or secrets?*

    vi. Appears indifferent to praise or criticism: *When other people praise or criticize you, do you find that it does not affect you?*

    vii. Shows emotional coldness or detachment: *Do you rarely experience strong emotions like anger or joy? Do you rarely reciprocate gestures or facial expressions like smiles or nods?*

b. Exclusion: If the disturbance occurs exclusively in the course of a psychotic disorder, a bipolar or depressive disorder with psychotic features, or autism spectrum disorder, or is a physiological effect of another medical condition, do not make the diagnosis.

3. Schizotypal Personality Disorder

a. Inclusion: Requires a pervasive pattern of social and interpersonal deficits marked by acute discomfort with, and reduced capacity for, close relationships as well as by cognitive or perceptual distortions or eccentricities, as indicated by at least <u>five</u> of the following manifestations.

i. Ideas of reference: *Does it often feel as though other people are talking about you or watching you?*

ii. Odd beliefs or magical thinking: *Are you very superstitious? Are you preoccupied with paranormal or magical phenomena? Do you have special powers to sense events before they happen or to read the thoughts of other people?*

iii. Unusual perceptual experiences: *Do you sometimes have the sense that another person, whom other people cannot see, is present and speaking with you?*

iv. Odd thinking and speech: *Do other people ever tell you that the things you say, or the way you say them, are unusual or even inappropriate?*

v. Suspiciousness or paranoia: *Do you frequently suspect that other people are exploiting, harming, or deceiving you?*

vi. Inappropriate or constricted affect: *Do you notice that your emotional experiences and expressions stay within a narrow range and do not change much over time? Have other people told you that you do not respond to emotionally provocative situations as they expect?*

vii. Odd or eccentric appearance or behavior: *Do other people ever respond to you as if your behavior or appearance was odd or bizarre?*

viii. Lacks close friends and confidants: *Other than your immediate family, do you find that you do not have close friends or people with whom you share personal matters or secrets?*

ix. Excessive social anxiety: *Are you usually worried or anxious in social settings, especially when around unfamiliar people?*

b. Exclusion: If the disturbance occurs exclusively in the course of a psychotic disorder, a bipolar or depressive disorder with psychotic features, or an autism spectrum disorder, do not make the diagnosis.

4. Antisocial Personality Disorder

   a. Inclusion: Requires a pervasive pattern of disregard for and violation of the rights of others, as indicated by at least <u>three</u> of the following manifestations.

      i. Repeatedly performing acts that are grounds for arrest: *Have you repeatedly destroyed or stolen the property of other people, harassed other people, or done other things that could have gotten you arrested?*

      ii. Deceitfulness: *Do you often misrepresent yourself by claiming accomplishments, qualities, or identities that are not your own? Do you often deceive other people for pleasure or financial gain?*

      iii. Impulsivity: *Do you often struggle to formulate and follow a plan? Do you often act on the spur of the moment, without a plan or consideration of the consequences?*

      iv. Aggressiveness resulting in assaults: *Are you often so grumpy or irritable that you frequently confront or even attack other people? Have you ever attacked someone or been in physical fights that did not begin as self-defense?*

      v. Reckless disregard for safety: *Do you often engage in dangerous, risky, and potentially self-damaging activities with little thought to the consequences for yourself or others?*

      vi. Consistent irresponsibility: *When you enter into agreements or make promises, do you often disregard and fail to follow through on your commitments? When you have familial obligations and financial debts, do you often disregard them?*

      vii. Lack of remorse: *Are you rarely concerned about the feelings, needs, or suffering of other people? If you have ever hurt or mistreated someone else, did you feel very little regret or remorse after doing so?*

   b. Inclusion: Evidence of conduct disorder with onset before the age of 15 years.

   c. Exclusion: If the disturbance occurs exclusively in the course of a psychotic or bipolar disorder, do not make the diagnosis.

5. Borderline Personality Disorder

   a. Inclusion: Requires a pervasive pattern of instability of interpersonal relationships, self-image, and affects, and marked impulsivity, as indicated by at least <u>five</u> of the following manifestations.

      i. Frantic efforts to avoid abandonment: *When you sense that someone close to you is going to abandon you, do you undertake emotional or even frantic efforts to keep them from leaving you?*

      ii. Unstable interpersonal relationships: *Are most of your close relationships intense and unstable? Do you alternate between feeling as though the people in your life are really good and really bad?*

      iii. Identity disturbance: *Do you have a very unstable or poorly developed sense of who you are? Do your aspirations, goals, opinions, and values change suddenly and frequently?*

      iv. Self-damaging impulsivity in at least two areas that are not suicidal or self-mutilating behavior: *Do you often act on the spur of the moment, without a plan or consideration for the outcome? Do you frequently engage in dangerous, risky, and potentially self-damaging activities without regard to their consequences?*

      v. Parasuicidal or suicidal behavior: *Do you frequently threaten to harm yourself or even kill yourself? Have you made recurrent attempts to hurt, harm, or kill yourself?*

      vi. Affective instability: *Are your emotions easily aroused or intense? Do you often have intense feelings of sadness, annoyance, or worry that usually only last a few hours and never more than a few days?*

      vii. Chronic emptiness: *Do you chronically feel empty?*

      viii. Anger: *Do you often experience intense anger, often much stronger than the event or circumstance that triggered it, and frequently lose your temper?*

      ix. Transient paranoia or dissociation: *At times of stress, do you ever feel like other people are conspiring against you or that you are an outside observer of your own mind, thoughts, feelings, and body?*

6. Histrionic Personality Disorder

   a. Inclusion: Requires a pervasive pattern of excessive emotionality and attention seeking, as indicated by at least <u>five</u> of the following manifestations.

    i. Uncomfortable when not the center of attention: *Do you usually feel uncomfortable or unappreciated when you are not the center of attention?*

    ii. Seductive or provocative behavior: *Do you flirt with most of the people you meet, even if you are not attracted to them?*

    iii. Shifting and shallow emotions: *When you express emotions or feelings, do they change rapidly? Have other people told you that your emotions seem to have little depth or to be insincere?*

    iv. Uses appearance to draw attention: *Do you usually "dress to impress," spending your time and energy on your clothes and appearance so you can draw attention to yourself?*

    v. Impressionistic and vague speech: *Do other people ever tell you that you have strong opinions but that they find it hard to understand the underlying reasons for your opinions?*

    vi. Dramatic or exaggerated emotions: *Are you a very expressive or even dramatic person? Have your friends or family repeatedly told you that you embarrassed them with your public displays of emotion?*

    vii. Suggestible: *Do you frequently change your opinions and feelings based on the people around you or the people you admire?*

    viii. Considers relationships more intimate than they are: *Do you often feel close to people early in a relationship and share personal details of your life? Have you been hurt by relationships that you thought were more serious or intimate than the other person did?*

7. Narcissistic Personality Disorder

  a. Inclusion: Requires a pervasive pattern of grandiosity (in fantasy or behavior), need for admiration, and lack of empathy, as indicated by at least <u>five</u> of the following manifestations.

    i. Grandiose sense of self-importance: *Would you describe yourself and your accomplishments as so special and unique that they set you apart from your peers?*

    ii. Preoccupied with fantasies of unlimited success: *When you imagine the life of your dreams, do you think a lot about having unlimited success, limitless power, unparalleled brilliance, remarkable beauty, or supreme love?*

   iii. High-status understanding: *Are your abilities and needs so special that you feel as though you should associate only with gifted people or institutions? Do you feel that only unique or gifted people are capable of understanding you?*

   iv. Requires excessive admiration: *Do you often feel offended if people you respect do not give you the admiration you deserve?*

   v. Entitlement: *Do you often get annoyed or irritated when people do not follow your wishes or give you the treatment you deserve?*

   vi. Exploitative: *Are you good at getting people to do what you want? Do you take advantage of people to get what you deserve?*

   vii. Lacks empathy: *Do you find it hard to recognize or identify with the feelings and needs of other people?*

   viii. Envious: *Do other people really envy you or your life? Do you spend a lot of time envying other people or their lives?*

   ix. Arrogant behaviors or attitudes: *Have other people ever told you that you acted haughty, patronizing, or arrogant?*

8. Avoidant Personality Disorder

   a. Inclusion: Requires a pervasive pattern of social inhibition, feelings of inadequacy, and hypersensitivity to negative evaluations, as indicated by at least <u>four</u> of the following manifestations.

     i. Avoids occupational activities involving interpersonal contact: *Do you often avoid school or work activities that involve a lot of contact with other people because you fear they will criticize or reject you?*

     ii. Needs assurance before getting involved with other people: *Do you avoid meeting new people unless you are certain they like you and accept you without criticism?*

     iii. Fear of being shamed limits intimate relationships: *In your close relationships, are you usually cautious or restrained because you fear being shamed or ridiculed?*

     iv. Preoccupied with criticism in social situations: *In social situations, do you spend a great deal of time worrying that other people will criticize or reject you?*

     v. Inadequacy inhibits interpersonal situations: *In new relationships, are you usually shy, quiet, or inhibited because you fear that other people will find you inadequate or unsuitable?*

     vi. Negative self-perception: *Do you perceive yourself to be socially inept, personally unappealing, or inferior to others?*

    vii. Reluctant to take risks: *Are you usually reluctant to take personal risks or engage in any new activities because you fear you will be embarrassed?*

9. Dependent Personality Disorder

    a. Inclusion: Requires a pervasive and excessive need to be taken care of that leads to submissive and clinging behavior and fears of separation, as indicated by at least <u>five</u> of the following manifestations.

        i. Struggles to make everyday decisions without reassurance: *Do you struggle to make everyday decisions like what to eat or wear without advice and reassurance from other people?*

        ii. Needs others to assume responsibility: *Do you prefer to let someone else take responsibility for the major decisions in your life like where to live, the kind of work you do, and whom you befriend?*

        iii. Struggles to disagree: *Do you find it really hard to disagree with the people you count on because you fear they will disapprove or withdraw their support of you?*

        iv. Struggles to initiate: *Do you usually lack the self-confidence to start a new project or do things independently?*

        v. Excessive lengths to obtain support: *Do you go to great lengths to receive care and support from other people, even volunteering to do things that you find unpleasant?*

        vi. Feels helpless when alone: *When you are alone, do you often feel uncomfortable or even helpless because you fear being unable to care for yourself?*

        vii. Urgently seeks relationships: *After a close relationship ends, do you urgently seek another relationship in which you can receive the care and support you need?*

        viii. Preoccupied with fears of being alone: *Do you spend a great deal of time worrying about being left alone with no one to care for you?*

10. Obsessive-Compulsive Personality Disorder

    a. Inclusion: Requires a pervasive pattern of preoccupation with orderliness, perfectionism, and mental and interpersonal control, at the expense of flexibility, openness, and efficiency, as indicated by at least <u>four</u> of the following manifestations.

        i. Preoccupation with order interferes with the point of the activity: *Do you often find that you are so focused on* the details, rules, lists, order, organization, or schedules for an activity that you lose the essential point of the activity?

ii. Perfectionism interferes with task completion: *Are you often unable to complete projects because you cannot meet the high standards you set for yourself?*

iii. Devoted to work at the expense of friendships: *Do you devote so much time and energy to your work that you have little time for friendships or recreational activities?*

iv. Scrupulosity: *Do other people who share your cultural or religious identification ever tell you that they find you too strict or too concerned with not doing something wrong? Do you aspire to moral standards that are so high that it is difficult for you to realize your goals?*

v. Unable to discard worn-out objects: *Do you often find it hard to discard worn-out or worthless objects even when they have no sentimental value?*

vi. Reluctant to give up control of tasks: *Do you find it hard to work with other people or delegate tasks because you fear they will not do things the way you would?*

vii. Miserly: *Do you usually find it hard to spend money on yourself or other people? Do you maintain a standard of living well below what you can afford so you can save money for a catastrophe?*

viii. Rigidity: *Does your need to be right, or to not change your position, frequently make it difficult to make and maintain relationships with other people?*

11. Alternative:

a. If a person exhibits a persistent personality disturbance that represents a change from their previous characteristic personality pattern and there is evidence that the disturbance is the direct consequence of another medical condition, consider personality change due to another medical condition (full criteria and multiple specifiers are in DSM-5-TR, pp. 775–776). If the diagnosis is better explained by another mental disorder, occurs exclusively during an episode of delirium, or does not cause clinically significant distress or impairment, do not make the diagnosis.

b. If a person exhibits symptoms characteristic of a personality disorder that cause clinically significant distress or impairment but do not meet full criteria for a specific personality disorder, consider unspecified personality disorder (see DSM-5-TR, p. 778). If you wish to communicate the specific reason that the presentation does not meet the criteria for a specific personality disorder, consider other specified personality disorder (see DSM-5-TR, p. 778).

Paraphilic Disorders

DSM-5-TR pp. 779–801

Screening question: *Are there any particular urges, fantasies, or behaviors that repeatedly cause you to feel intensely aroused and worry you or other people?*

If yes, ask: *Has satisfying these fantasies or urges put you or someone else at harm?* OR *Have you acted on these fantasies or urges with someone who did not want to be involved?*

- If yes, proceed to paraphilic disorder criteria.

1. Paraphilic Disorders
   a. Inclusion: Requires a paraphilia, which is any intense and persistent sexual interest other than sexual interest in genital stimulation with mature, consenting partners. The paraphilia must be intense and persistent for at least 6 months and must be currently causing distress or impairment in the individual, or entail personal harm or risk of harm to others, to qualify as disordered.
      i. Paraphilia: *Different people are differently aroused. I am going to read a list of fantasies, urges, and behaviors and would like you to tell me if you experience any of these frequently and recurrently.*
         - Voyeuristic disorder: *Are you intensely aroused by watching people who do not know that you are watching while they are naked, disrobing, or engaging in sexual activity?*
         - Exhibitionistic disorder: *Are you intensely aroused by the thought of exposing your genitals to a person who does not want to be exposed to them?*
         - Frotteuristic disorder: *Are you intensely aroused by the thought of touching or rubbing against a nonconsenting person?*
         - Sexual masochism disorder: *Are you intensely aroused by the thought of being humiliated, bound, beaten, or otherwise made to suffer?*

- Sexual sadism disorder: *Are you intensely aroused by the physical or psychological suffering of another person?*
- Pedophilic disorder: *Are you intensely aroused by sexual activity with prepubescent or pubescent children?*
- Fetishistic disorder: *Are you intensely aroused by nonliving objects other than clothes used in cross-dressing or devices designed for genital stimulation? Are you intensely aroused by specific nongenital body parts like feet, toes, or hair?*
- Transvestic disorder: *Are you intensely aroused by cross-dressing?*

b. Exclusions

   i. For the diagnosis of voyeuristic disorder, the person experiencing the arousal and/or acting on the urges must be at least 18 years of age.
   ii. For the diagnosis of pedophilic disorder, the person must be at least 16 years of age and at least 5 years older than the child or children who are the object(s) of arousal.
   iii. For the diagnosis of fetishistic disorder, the object of arousal cannot include clothing used in cross-dressing or objects specifically designed for tactile genital stimulation, such as a vibrator.

c. Modifiers

   i. Course specifiers common to paraphilic disorders (do not apply to pedophilic disorder)

      - In a controlled environment
      - In full remission (no recurring behavior or distress or impairment for at least 5 years while in an uncontrolled environment)

   ii. Exhibitionistic disorder subtypes

      - Sexually aroused by exposing genitals to prepubertal children
      - Sexually aroused by exposing genitals to physically mature individuals
      - Sexually aroused by exposing genitals to prepubertal children and to physically mature individuals

iii. Sexual masochism disorder specifier
- With asphyxiophilia (i.e., sexually aroused by restriction of breathing)

iv. Pedophilic disorder subtypes
- Exclusive type (attracted only to children)
- Nonexclusive type

v. Pedophilic disorder specifiers
- Sexually attracted to males
- Sexually attracted to females
- Sexually attracted to both
- Limited to incest

vi. Fetishistic disorder specifiers
- Body part(s)
- Nonliving object(s)
- Other

vii. Transvestic disorder specifiers
- With fetishism (sexually aroused by fabrics, materials, or garments)
- With autogynephilia (sexually aroused by thought or image of self as a woman)

d. Alternatives: If a person endorses a paraphilia that is not included in this list, consider unspecified paraphilic disorder (see DSM-5-TR, p. 801). If you wish to communicate the specific reason a person's presentation does not meet full criteria for a disorder above, consider other specified paraphilic disorder (see DSM-5-TR, p. 801). DSM-5-TR includes a partial list of paraphilias that can occur within a paraphilic disorder: telephone scatologia disorder (obscene phone calls), necrophilic disorder (corpses), zoophilic disorder (animals), coprophilic disorder (feces), klismaphilic disorder (enemas), and urophilic disorder (urine).

Medication-Induced Movement Disorders and Other Adverse Effects of Medication

DSM-5-TR pp. 807–819

ICD-10-CM code	Description
G21.11	Antipsychotic medication and other dopamine receptor blocking agent–induced parkinsonism
G21.19	Other medication-induced parkinsonism
G21.0	Neuroleptic malignant syndrome
G24.02	Medication-induced acute dystonia
G25.71	Medication-induced acute akathisia
G24.01	Tardive dyskinesia
G24.09	Tardive dystonia
G25.71	Tardive akathisia
G25.1	Medication-induced postural tremor
G25.79	Other medication-induced movement disorder
	Antidepressant discontinuation syndrome
T43.205A	Initial encounter
T43.205D	Subsequent encounter
T43.205S	Sequelae
	Other adverse effect of medication
T50.905A	Initial encounter
T50.905D	Subsequent encounter
T50.905S	Sequelae

Other Conditions That May Be a Focus of Clinical Attention

DSM-5-TR pp. 821–836

A patient's mental disorder is affected by the other conditions and any psychosocial or environmental problems they have.

To assist a clinician addressing the other conditions that alter the diagnosis, course, prognosis, and treatment of a patient's mental disorder, DSM-5-TR provides a selected list of conditions and problems drawn from ICD-10-CM (usually Z codes). A condition or problem listed below may be coded if it is initiated or exacerbated by a mental disorder, is a reason for the current visit, constitutes a problem that must be considered for the overall management, or otherwise helps explain the need for a test, procedure, or treatment.

Conditions and problems from this list may also be included in the medical record as useful information on circumstances that may affect the patient's care, regardless of their relevance to the current visit. The conditions and problems listed in this chapter are not mental disorders. Their inclusion in DSM-5-TR is meant to draw attention to the scope of additional issues that are encountered in routine clinical practice and to provide a systematic listing that may be useful to clinicians in documenting these issues.

TABLE 6–1. Other Conditions That May Be a Focus of Clinical Attention

---

Suicidal Behavior and Nonsuicidal Self-Injury

Suicidal Behavior

	Current Suicidal Behavior
T14.91A	Initial encounter
T14.91D	Subsequent encounter
Z91.51	History of Suicidal Behavior

Nonsuicidal Self-Injury

R45.88	Current Nonsuicidal Self-Injury
Z91.52	History of Nonsuicidal Self-Injury

Abuse and Neglect

Child Maltreatment and Neglect Problems

Child Physical Abuse

	Child Physical Abuse, Confirmed
T74.12XA	Initial encounter
T74.12XD	Subsequent encounter
	Child Physical Abuse, Suspected
T76.12XA	Initial encounter
T76.12XD	Subsequent encounter

TABLE 6–1. Other Conditions That May Be a Focus of Clinical Attention *(continued)*

Other Circumstances Related to Child Physical Abuse

Z69.010	Encounter for mental health services for victim of child physical abuse by parent
Z69.020	Encounter for mental health services for victim of nonparental child physical abuse
Z62.810	Personal history (past history) of physical abuse in childhood
Z69.011	Encounter for mental health services for perpetrator of parental child physical abuse
Z69.021	Encounter for mental health services for perpetrator of nonparental child physical abuse

Child Sexual Abuse

Child Sexual Abuse, Confirmed

T74.22XA	Initial encounter
T74.22XD	Subsequent encounter

Child Sexual Abuse, Suspected

T76.22XA	Initial encounter
T76.22XD	Subsequent encounter

Other Circumstances Related to Child Sexual Abuse

Z69.010	Encounter for mental health services for victim of child sexual abuse by parent
Z69.020	Encounter for mental health services for victim of nonparental child sexual abuse
Z62.810	Personal history (past history) of sexual abuse in childhood
Z69.011	Encounter for mental health services for perpetrator of parental child sexual abuse
Z69.021	Encounter for mental health services for perpetrator of nonparental child sexual abuse

Child Neglect

Child Neglect, Confirmed

T74.02XA	Initial encounter
T74.02XD	Subsequent encounter

Child Neglect, Suspected

T76.02XA	Initial encounter
T76.02XD	Subsequent encounter

Other Circumstances Related to Child Neglect

Z69.010 Encounter for mental health services for victim
of child neglect by parent

Z69.020 Encounter for mental health services for victim
of nonparental child neglect

Z62.812 Personal history (past history) of neglect in
childhood

Z69.011 Encounter for mental health services for
perpetrator of parental child neglect

Z69.021 Encounter for mental health services for
perpetrator of nonparental child neglect

Child Psychological Abuse

Child Psychological Abuse, Confirmed

T74.32XA Initial encounter

T74.32XD Subsequent encounter

Child Psychological Abuse, Suspected

T76.32XA Initial encounter

T76.32XD Subsequent encounter

*Other Circumstances Related to Child Psychological
Abuse*

Z69.010 Encounter for mental health services for victim
of child psychological abuse by parent

Z69.020 Encounter for mental health services for victim
of nonparental child psychological abuse

Z62.811 Personal history (past history) of psychological
abuse in childhood

Z69.011 Encounter for mental health services for
perpetrator of parental child psychological
abuse

Z69.021 Encounter for mental health services for
perpetrator of nonparental child psychological
abuse

TABLE 6–1. Other Conditions That May Be a Focus of Clinical Attention *(continued)*

Adult Maltreatment and Neglect Problems

Spouse or Partner Violence, Physical

        Spouse or Partner Violence, Physical, Confirmed

T74.11XA	Initial encounter
T74.11XD	Subsequent encounter

        Spouse or Partner Violence, Physical, Suspected

T76.11XA	Initial encounter
T76.11XD	Subsequent encounter

        Other Circumstances Related to Spouse or Partner Violence, Physical

Z69.11	Encounter for mental health services for victim of spouse or partner violence, physical
Z91.410	Personal history (past history) of spouse or partner violence, physical
Z69.12	Encounter for mental health services for perpetrator of spouse or partner violence, physical

Spouse or Partner Violence, Sexual

        Spouse or Partner Violence, Sexual, Confirmed

T74.21XA	Initial encounter
T74.21XD	Subsequent encounter

        Spouse or Partner Violence, Sexual, Suspected

T76.21XA	Initial encounter
T76.21XD	Subsequent encounter

        Other Circumstances Related to Spouse or Partner Violence, Sexual

Z69.81	Encounter for mental health services for victim of spouse or partner violence, sexual
Z91.410	Personal history (past history) of spouse or partner violence, sexual
Z69.12	Encounter for mental health services for perpetrator of spouse or partner violence, sexual

TABLE 6–1. Other Conditions That May Be a Focus of Clinical Attention *(continued)*

Spouse or Partner Neglect

          Spouse or Partner Neglect, Confirmed

T74.01XA   Initial encounter

T74.01XD   Subsequent encounter

          Spouse or Partner Neglect, Suspected

T76.01XA   Initial encounter

T76.01XD   Subsequent encounter

          Other Circumstances Related to Spouse or Partner Neglect

Z69.11   Encounter for mental health services for victim of spouse or partner neglect

Z91.412   Personal history (past history) of spouse or partner neglect

Z69.12   Encounter for mental health services for perpetrator of spouse or partner neglect

Spouse or Partner Abuse, Psychological

          Spouse or Partner Abuse, Psychological, Confirmed

T74.31XA   Initial encounter

T74.31XD   Subsequent encounter

          Spouse or Partner Abuse, Psychological, Suspected

T76.31XA   Initial encounter

T76.31XD   Subsequent encounter

          Other Circumstances Related to Spouse or Partner Abuse, Psychological

Z69.11   Encounter for mental health services for victim of spouse or partner psychological abuse

Z91.411   Personal history (past history) of spouse or partner psychological abuse

Z69.12   Encounter for mental health services for perpetrator of spouse or partner psychological abuse

TABLE 6–1. Other Conditions That May Be a Focus of Clinical Attention *(continued)*

Adult Abuse by Nonspouse or Nonpartner

	Adult Physical Abuse by Nonspouse or Nonpartner, Confirmed
T74.11XA	Initial encounter
T74.11XD	Subsequent encounter
	Adult Physical Abuse by Nonspouse or Nonpartner, Suspected
T76.11XA	Initial encounter
T76.11XD	Subsequent encounter
	Adult Sexual Abuse by Nonspouse or Nonpartner, Confirmed
T74.21XA	Initial encounter
T74.21XD	Subsequent encounter
	Adult Sexual Abuse by Nonspouse or Nonpartner, Suspected
T76.21XA	Initial encounter
T76.21XD	Subsequent encounter
	Adult Psychological Abuse by Nonspouse or Nonpartner, Confirmed
T74.31XA	Initial encounter
T74.31XD	Subsequent encounter
	Adult Psychological Abuse by Nonspouse or Nonpartner, Suspected
T76.31XA	Initial encounter
T76.31XD	Subsequent encounter
	Other Circumstances Related to Adult Abuse by Nonspouse or Nonpartner
Z69.81	Encounter for mental health services for victim of nonspousal or nonpartner adult abuse
Z69.82	Encounter for mental health services for perpetrator of nonspousal or nonpartner adult abuse

TABLE 6–1. Other Conditions That May Be a Focus of Clinical Attention *(continued)*

Relational Problems

Parent-Child Relational Problem

Z62.820	Parent–Biological Child
Z62.821	Parent–Adopted Child
Z62.822	Parent–Foster Child
Z62.898	Other Caregiver–Child
Z62.891	Sibling Relational Problem
Z63.0	Relationship Distress With Spouse or Intimate Partner

Problems Related to the Family Environment

Z62.29	Upbringing Away From Parents
Z62.898	Child Affected by Parental Relationship Distress
Z63.5	Disruption of Family by Separation or Divorce
Z63.8	High Expressed Emotion Level Within Family

Educational Problems

Z55.0	Illiteracy and Low-Level Literacy
Z55.1	Schooling Unavailable and Unattainable
Z55.2	Failed School Examinations
Z55.3	Underachievement in School
Z55.4	Educational Maladjustment and Discord With Teachers and Classmates
Z55.8	Problems Related to Inadequate Teaching
Z55.9	Other Problems Related to Education and Literacy

Occupational Problems

Z56.82	Problem Related to Current Military Deployment Status
Z56.0	Unemployment
Z56.1	Change of Job
Z56.2	Threat of Job Loss
Z56.3	Stressful Work Schedule
Z56.4	Discord With Boss and Workmates
Z56.5	Uncongenial Work Environment
Z56.6	Other Physical and Mental Strain Related to Work
Z56.81	Sexual Harassment on the Job
Z56.9	Other Problem Related to Employment

TABLE 6–1. Other Conditions That May Be a Focus of Clinical Attention *(continued)*

Housing Problems

Z59.01	Sheltered Homelessness
Z59.02	Unsheltered Homelessness
Z59.1	Inadequate Housing
Z59.2	Discord With Neighbor, Lodger, or Landlord
Z59.3	Problem Related to Living in a Residential Institution
Z59.9	Other Housing Problem

Economic Problems

Z59.41	Food Insecurity
Z58.6	Lack of Safe Drinking Water
Z59.5	Extreme Poverty
Z59.6	Low Income
Z59.7	Insufficient Social Insurance or Welfare Support
Z59.9	Other Economic Problem

Problems Related to the Social Environment

Z60.2	Problem Related to Living Alone
Z60.3	Acculturation Difficulty
Z60.4	Social Exclusion or Rejection
Z60.5	Target of (Perceived) Adverse Discrimination or Persecution
Z60.9	Other Problem Related to Social Environment

Problems Related to Interaction With the Legal System

Z65.0	Conviction in Civil or Criminal Proceedings Without Imprisonment
Z65.1	Imprisonment or Other Incarceration
Z65.2	Problems Related to Release From Prison
Z65.3	Problems Related to Other Legal Circumstances

TABLE 6–1. Other Conditions That May Be a Focus of Clinical Attention *(continued)*

Problems Related to Other Psychosocial, Personal, and Environmental Circumstances

Z72.9	Problem Related to Lifestyle
Z64.0	Problems Related to Unwanted Pregnancy
Z64.1	Problems Related to Multiparity
Z64.4	Discord With Social Service Provider, Including Probation Officer, Case Manager, or Social Services Worker
Z65.4	Victim of Crime
Z65.4	Victim of Terrorism or Torture
Z65.5	Exposure to Disaster, War, or Other Hostilities

Problems Related to Access to Medical and Other Health Care

Z75.3	Unavailability or Inaccessibility of Health Care Facilities
Z75.4	Unavailability or Inaccessibility of Other Helping Agencies

Circumstances of Personal History

Z91.49	Personal History of Psychological Trauma
Z91.82	Personal History of Military Deployment

Other Health Service Encounters for Counseling and Medical Advice

Z31.5	Genetic Counseling
Z70.9	Sex Counseling
Z71.3	Dietary Counseling
Z71.9	Other Counseling or Consultation

TABLE 6–1.	Other Conditions That May Be a Focus of Clinical Attention *(continued)*

Additional Conditions or Problems That May Be a Focus of Clinical Attention

Z91.83	Wandering Associated With a Mental Disorder
Z63.4	Uncomplicated Bereavement
Z60.0	Phase of Life Problem
Z65.8	Religious or Spiritual Problem
Z72.811	Adult Antisocial Behavior
Z72.810	Child or Adolescent Antisocial Behavior
Z91.19	Nonadherence to Medical Treatment
E66.9	Overweight or Obesity
Z76.5	Malingering
R41.81	Age-Related Cognitive Decline
R41.83	Borderline Intellectual Functioning

SECTION III

Chapter 7

A Brief Version of DSM-5-TR

Diagnosis	Criteria/Time	Symptoms
Neurodevelopmental disorders		
Autism spectrum disorder	All 3 in multiple contexts, beginning in early childhood *AND*	Deficits in social-emotional reciprocity; deficits in nonverbal communicative behaviors; deficits in developing and maintaining relationships
	≥2	Stereotyped or repetitive motor movements, use of objects, or speech; inflexible adherence to routines or excessive resistance to change; highly restricted, fixated interests of abnormal intensity or focus; hyperreactivity or hyporeactivity to sensory input
Attention-deficit/ hyperactivity disorder	≥6 for ≥6 months *OR*	Inattention: makes careless mistakes; cannot sustain attention; does not seem to listen; often does not follow through; struggles to organize tasks; dislikes sustained mental effort; loses objects necessary for tasks; distracted by extraneous stimuli; forgetful in daily activities
	≥6 for ≥6 months	Hyperactivity/impulsivity: fidgets; leaves seat when sitting is expected; runs or climbs when inappropriate; unable to remain quiet; on the go; talks excessively; blurts out answers; cannot wait turn; interrupts; acts without thinking

Diagnosis	Criteria/Time	Symptoms
Schizophrenia spectrum and other psychotic disorders		
Schizophrenia	≥2 for ≥1 month *AND*	Delusions; hallucinations; disorganized speech; grossly disorganized or catatonic behavior; negative symptoms (at least one symptom is delusions, hallucinations, or disorganized speech)
	≥6 months	Continuous signs of disturbance
Schizoaffective disorder		Criteria for schizophrenia
	≥50% of the time *AND*	Also experiences major depressive or manic episodes
	≥2 weeks	Delusions or hallucinations without depressive or manic episodes

Diagnosis	Criteria/Time	Symptoms
Bipolar and related disorders		
Bipolar I disorder	≥1 week (or any duration if hospitalized) *AND* ≥3	Mania: abnormally, persistently elevated or irritable mood and increased activity or energy Inflated self-esteem or grandiosity; decreased need for sleep; pressured speech; flight of ideas or racing thoughts; distractibility; increase in goal-directed activity; excessive involvement in activities with high potential for painful consequences
Bipolar II disorder	≥4 days *AND* ≥3	Hypomania: abnormally, persistently elevated or irritable mood and increased activity or energy Inflated self-esteem or grandiosity; decreased need for sleep; pressured speech; flight of ideas or racing thoughts; distractibility; increased goal-directed activity; excessive involvement in activities with high potential for painful consequences *without* psychosis or hospitalization

Diagnosis	Criteria/Time	Symptoms
Depressive disorders		
Major depressive disorder	≥1 for ≥2 weeks *AND*	Depressed mood most of the day; marked loss of interest in activities or pleasure (anhedonia)
	≥4 for ≥2 weeks	Significant unintentional weight loss or decreased appetite; insomnia/hypersomnia; psychomotor agitation/retardation; fatigue or loss of energy; worthlessness or excessive guilt; decreased ability to concentrate; recurrent thoughts of death or suicide
Anxiety disorders		
Panic disorder	≥4 *AND*	Recurrent surges of intense fear or intense discomfort demonstrated by palpitations; sweating; trembling; shortness of breath; choking sensation; chest pain; nausea; dizziness; chills; paresthesias; derealization; fear of losing control or sanity; fear of death
	≥1 month	Persistent concern or worry *OR* Maladaptive change in behavior related to panic attacks
Generalized anxiety disorder	≥3	Restlessness; easily fatigued; difficulty concentrating; irritability; muscle tension; sleep disturbance
	≥6 months *AND*	Excessive anxiety and worry (apprehensive expectation) that is difficult to control

Diagnosis	Criteria/Time	Symptoms
Obsessive-compulsive and related disorders		
Obsessive-compulsive disorder	≥1 hour/day	Obsessions: recurrent and intrusive thoughts, urges, or images that a person attempts to ignore or suppress through compulsive acts *AND/OR* Compulsions: repetitive behaviors or mental acts to reduce distress
Trauma- and stressor-related disorders		
Posttraumatic stress disorder	*AND*	Exposure to actual or threatened death, serious injury, or sexual violence
	≥1 for ≥1 month *AND*	Intrusions: distressing memories; intrusive dreams; flashbacks; exposure to triggers causing distress; marked physiological reactions
	≥1 for ≥1 month	Avoidance: internal reminders; external reminders of trauma
	≥2 for ≥1 month *AND*	Negative symptoms: impaired memory of trauma; negative self-worth; pathological blame; negative emotions; decreased participation; detachment; emotional numbness
	≥2 for ≥1 month	Reactive arousal: irritability or aggression; recklessness; hypervigilance; exaggerated startle response; impaired concentration; sleep disturbance

Diagnosis	Criteria/Time	Symptoms
Neurocognitive disorders		
Delirium	Acute	Disturbance of attention with reduced environmental awareness; acute change from baseline, generally with fluctuating severity; cognitive disturbance
Major neurocognitive disorder	Insidious	Significant cognitive decline, ≥2 standard deviations (SDs) below normal, which interferes with independence
Mild neurocognitive disorder	Insidious	Minor cognitive decline, 1–2 SDs below normal, which does not interfere with independence (but may require greater effort, compensatory strategies, or accommodations to maintain level of functioning)

Chapter 8

Six Questions to a Differential Diagnosis

Since a person's mental distress can be explained
in multiple ways, a good clinician considers many diagnoses
when pursuing their explanation of a patient's distress (Feinstein 1967). In their investigations, a clinician systematically
considers at least six explanatory groups of possibilities. As a
clinician develops their clinical decision-making, it is helpful
to investigate these six possibilities sequentially to develop
their habit of reflecting upon what psychiatrist Kenneth Kendler
(2012, p. 377) calls "the dappled nature," the many and interre-
lated causes, of mental disorders. Clinicians interested in exploring further steps of differential diagnosis should read texts
specific to psychiatric evaluation (e.g. Chisolm and Lyketsos
2012) and the DSM-5-TR *Handbook of Differential Diagnosis* (First
2023).

Question 1: Could the Signs and Symptoms Be Intentionally Produced?

Always consider whether a patient might be intentionally producing findings, because an honest report of psychiatric symptoms and signs is the foundation for developing a fruitful
diagnosis and treatment plan. An honest report strengthens
the therapeutic alliance, while a dishonest report weakens the
therapeutic alliance. If intentionally produced findings are
associated with an obvious external award—such as money,
disability, or time off—consider the possibility of malingering.
Malingering may be concomitant with other medical and psychiatric diagnoses.

If intentionally produced findings are associated with the
desire to be perceived as ill or impaired, consider factitious
disorder.

A patient can also unconsciously produce signs or symptoms to resolve a psychological conflict, to validate their inability to function socially, or as an attempt to secure assistance, such as the sick role, disability, or supported employment. In these situations, consider one of the somatic symptom and related disorders.

Question 2: Are the Signs and Symptoms Related to Substances?

The variety of substances that people use and misuse is remarkable, as are the clinical effects of substance use. People can experience mental distress during substance use, intoxication, and withdrawal. When you seek the cause of a patient's distress, always consider drugs of abuse, as well as prescription, over-the-counter, and herbal medicines or products. People often underreport their use of substances, so consider these possibilities:

- Substances may directly cause a patient's psychiatric signs and symptoms.
- A patient may use substances because of a mental disorder and its sequelae.
- A patient may use substances and experience psychiatric signs and symptoms, but the substance use and the signs and symptoms are unrelated.

Question 3: Are the Signs and Symptoms Related to Another Medical Condition?

A patient can present with another medical condition that mimics psychiatric signs and symptoms. Sometimes, presentation with these findings is a sentinel event that occurs in advance of the other stigmata of a medical condition. Alternatively, a patient may develop psychiatric signs and symptoms years after presentation for another medical condition. Clues that another medical condition may be related to a mental disorder include an atypical presentation, abnormal age at onset, and abnormal course. Consider these possibilities:

- Another medical condition may directly alter the patient's psychiatric signs and symptoms.
- Another medical condition may indirectly alter the patient's psychiatric signs and symptoms, as through a psychological mechanism.
- The treatment for another medical condition may directly alter the patient's psychiatric signs and symptoms.
- A mental disorder, or its treatment, may cause or exacerbate another medical condition.
- A patient may have a mental disorder and another medical condition, but they are causally unrelated.

Question 4: Are the Signs and Symptoms Related to a Developmental or Caregiver Conflict?

If you are evaluating a young child, your diagnostic interview should include formal developmental testing, a skill reviewed elsewhere (Hilt and Nussbaum 2016). Even when you are interviewing older children, adolescents, and adults, however, you should consider a patient's developmental stage, which can be quite different from the developmental stage you would expect based on their age, background, and education (Wang and Nussbaum 2017). A thorough social history will give you a sense of how a patient's current behavior relates to their usual behavior, but it is also useful to observe how your patient communicates and behaves, and compare their communication and behavior with those appropriate for their age.

Human beings are, in the words of the philosopher Alasdair MacIntyre, "dependent rational animals," because we depend upon "particular others for protection and sustenance" (MacIntyre 2012, p. 1). This dependence is acute for children, adolescents, the elderly, and many people with serious mental illnesses. By degrees of ability, age, development, impairment, and temperament, people depend upon caregivers. Caregivers can aid or injure a patient. Observe how a patient does (or does not) speak about the caregivers in their life, either directly or through transitional objects that embody psychological needs.

As you observe, consider these possibilities about why a patient may experience mental distress:

- They may be experiencing a transient regression in response to a particular event.
- They may be employing an immature defense mechanism, which may indicate a personality trait or disorder.
- They may be experiencing a developmental conflict in a particular relationship.
- They may have a developmental delay.
- They may have communication difficulties or cultural differences with a caregiver.
- They may have been (or are being) abused, neglected, or otherwise harmed by a caregiver.
- Their caregiver may be experiencing mental distress, resulting in the caregiver unintentionally worsening a patient's signs or symptoms.

Question 5: Are the Signs and Symptoms Related to a Mental Disorder?

DSM-5-TR diagnoses are summaries of information that allow you to categorize the experiences of a distressed person and to communicate with the other professionals caring for that person. A good clinician relies on the predominant symptomatology to support their diagnosis. DSM-5-TR seeks parsimony, but diagnoses are not mutually exclusive, so consider these possibilities:

- Condition A may predispose a patient to Condition B and vice versa.
- An underlying condition, such as a genetic predisposition, may make a patient susceptible to both Conditions A and B.
- A mediating factor, such as alterations in reward systems, may influence susceptibility to both Conditions A and B.
- Conditions A and B may be part of a more complex and unified syndrome that has been artificially split in the diagnostic system.
- The relationship between Conditions A and B may be artificially enhanced by overlaps in the diagnostic criteria.
- The comorbidity between Conditions A and B may be coincidental.

Question 6: Could It Be That No Mental Disorder Is Present?

"Normality" covers a wide range of behaviors and thoughts that vary across cultural groups and developmental stages. In DSM-5-TR, a mental disorder causes a "clinically significant disturbance in an individual's cognitions, emotion regulation, or behavior that reflects a dysfunction in the psychological, biological, or developmental processes underlying mental functioning" (American Psychiatric Association 2022, p. 14). When a patient's symptoms and presentation cause clinically significant distress or impairment without fulfilling the criteria for a specific mental disorder, consider alternatives:

- An *other specified* diagnosis, where a practitioner specifies why a patient's experience does not meet the criteria of a specific diagnosis.
- An *unspecified* diagnosis, where a practitioner does not specify why a patient's experience does not meet the criteria of a specific diagnosis. (This diagnosis implies that you presently have insufficient information to make an other specified diagnosis.)
- No psychiatric diagnosis at all. Many people live with one, two, or even several signs or symptoms of mental illness without meeting criteria for any DSM-5-TR mental disorder. After all, the boundaries between normality and abnormality are determined through the exercise of a clinician's experienced judgment and a culture's shifting sanctions.

Chapter 9

A Mental Status Examination: With Essential Psychiatric Glossary

A comprehensive mental status examination begins with a patient's outer appearances and progressively proceeds into their interior life. A clinician must carefully observe and thoughtfully question a patient, all the while keeping in mind cultural context, developmental stage, and educational level. To describe their findings, clinicians use a specialized language, which can be learned in psychiatric glossaries (Shahrokh et al. 2011) and the appendix to DSM-5-TR. A clinician can organize their experience of a patient's mental state using their own version of the format outlined below, which includes definitions for the essential terms for the mental status examination.

Appearance

Describe how the patient appears, which may include:

- Ability to make and maintain eye contact
- Appropriateness to situation
- Attitude toward interview
- Cleanliness
- Dress
- Grooming
- Habitus (general constitution and physical build)
- Posture

Behavior

Document the patient's behaviors, which may include:

- Ability to relate socially during your encounter
- Ambulatory status and, if possible, gait
- Catalepsy (maintenance of any physical position after being moved by examiner)
- Posturing (striking a pose and maintaining it)
- Drooling
- Mannerisms (unnecessary behaviors that are part of goal-directed behaviors)
- Presence of waxy flexibility (resistance of limbs to passive motion that improves with ongoing movement)
- Psychomotor agitation (excessive physical activity accompanied by inner tension)
- Psychomotor retardation (generalized slowing of cognitive, emotional, or physical responses)
- Stereotypies (non-goal-directed behaviors that are unusual in frequency, but not in the action itself)
- Signs of extrapyramidal symptoms or tardive dyskinesia
- Tics (involuntary, recurrent, nonrhythmic movement or vocalization)
- Tremor

Speech and Language

Describe or note (if present) the following characteristics of the patient's speech:

- Amount
- Latency (a pause of several seconds before responding to a question)
- Rate
- Rhythm
- Tone
- Volume

Document the following speech problems if present:

- Anomia (inability to name everyday objects)
- Dysnomia (inability to find words)

Emotion

Describe, if present, the following characteristics of a patient's emotional state:

- Affect (the emotional tone conveyed by speech and behaviors)
- Alexithymia (inability to describe or recognize one's own emotions)
- Appropriateness to situation
- Intensity
- Mood (the emotional state which is sustained throughout the encounter)
- Quality
- Range
- Stability

Thought Process

Describe how the patient thinks, and note any evidence of the following:

- Mutism (absence of speech)
- Alliteration
- Aphonia (ability to only whisper or croak)
- Thought blocking (sudden stops in the middle of a thought sequence)
- Clang association (words chosen purely for sound)
- Decreased latency of response (answering questions before you can finish asking them)
- Increased latency of response (long pauses before fairly normal speech)
- Derailment (running ideas into each other)
- Distractibility (being easily diverted by extraneous stimuli)
- Echolalia (repetition of words or statements of others)
- Flight of ideas (an illogical group of associations)
- Associations may be described as intact, circumstantial (providing unnecessary details but eventually answering a question), tangential (only initially responding to a question), or loose (providing responses unrelated to a question), or even word salad (random use of words)
- Neologisms (creation of words)

- Perseveration (repetition of the same motor or verbal response despite varied stimuli)
- Poverty of speech (brief, concrete responses with limited spontaneous speech)
- Push of speech (increased, rapid speech that is often loud and difficult to interrupt)
- Verbigeration (prolonged repetition of isolated words)

Thought Content

Comment on what a person discusses, including the presence of any of the following:

- Compulsions (irresistible impulses to perform a behavior)
- Obsessions (recurrent, persistent idea, image, or desire that dominates thought)
- Delusions (fixed, firm, false beliefs that are not part of a person's culture or religion)
- Grandiosity
- Guilt
- Hallucinations (perceptions of an absent stimulus)
- Illusions (misperceptions of an actual stimulus)
- Ideas of persecution
- Ideas of reference (perceptions that unrelated stimuli have a particular and unusual meaning specific to the person)
- Ideation, intent, or plan to harm self or others (suicidal, homicidal, or violent)
- Paranoia
- Passivity (submissive attitude to a perceived superior)
- Phobias (intense, unreasonable, specific fears)
- Thought insertion (perceiving that your thoughts are not your own, but inserted into your mind by others)
- Thought withdrawal (perception that others can take thoughts out of your mind without consent)

Cognition

Observe and comment on the patient's cognition and intellectual resources, including the following:

- Ability to abstract and to interpret culturally—and educationally—appropriate proverbs
- Ability to calculate
- Ability to read and write
- Fund of general information
- Learning style
- Impulse control
- Orientation
- Recent and remote memory

Insight/Judgment

Observe and comment on the patient's insight and judgment, including the following:

- Insight into their condition, especially as to whether they deny or appreciate their problem
- Judgment (mental ability to compare choices and make appropriate decisions) as related to presenting condition and age

Chapter 10

Mental Health Treatment Planning

A treatment plan can be understood as a regulatory requirement, one of the many chores of contemporary health care, or as a recipe for changing a patient's life.

The goal of any medical intervention is to help a patient effect a therapeutic change they cannot make on their own. Since the treatment plan is a mutually agreed upon recipe for doing so, it names what the patient needs to change, who will help them, and how they will make the change. A treatment plan will include a problem list, a list of measurable goals, and the best practices necessary to achieve them.

They are the what, who, and how of treatment plans.

Problem Lists

When a clinician evaluates a person in mental distress, their goal should be to create a therapeutic alliance, but the tangible result of an evaluation is a diagnosis. The treatment plan proceeds from an accurate diagnosis.

Diagnoses are organized into a problem list, a comprehensive and hierarchical catalog of the problems addressed during a current encounter.

The items on the list should be standardized to enable communication between clinicians. Individual clinicians account for mental distress and mental illness differently—some focus on dysfunctional neural circuits, others traumatic experiences, and still others maladaptive personality traits. When these clinicians wish to speak with each other, they need a standard list. DSM-5-TR is the consensus diagnostic system of contemporary psychiatry, our field's way for mental health clinicians to work together while we await a diagnostic system with greater validity.

The diagnoses generated by a DSM-5-TR interview are called *disorders*, rather than diseases or illnesses. Disorders are a kind of middle path between disease and illness because the term acknowledges the complex interplay of biological, social, cultural, and psychological factors in mental distress. Broadly speaking, a disorder simply means there is a disturbance in physical or psychological functioning. Using the "disorder" label to describe mental distress draws attention to how it impairs a person's function, suggests the complex interplay of events that result in mental distress, and implicitly acknowledges the limits of our knowledge about its causes (Kendler 2012). Since the field does not yet know enough to be more precise, the ongoing use of disorder in our diagnostic systems is an opportunity for humility and a spur to further study, but also a way to communicate together about a patient's experiences.

For DSM-5-TR to work, practitioners need to diagnose specific disorders. Standardization does not work without specificity. Imagine a recipe that asks you to add "a serving of fat." Someone following the recipe would have to interpret the recipe, asking if the author of the recipe meant, say, a spoonful of bacon drippings or a half-cup of coconut oil? Each is possible but results in a different dish; the recipe becomes more of a personal interpretation than a communal instruction. Similarly, practitioners should recognize that characterizing a person as having "an unspecified mental disorder" inadequately communicates the precise nature of the patient's illness to other practitioners.

A good clinician selects the most specific diagnosis for which a patient qualifies. If a clinician believes a grandmother is depressed, they determine not only if her depression constitutes a major depressive episode but if it is a single or recurrent episode, with or without psychotic features, and its degree of severity. This level of specificity enables communication with other clinicians and informs their treatment. Another clinician will know that there are different ways to treat a depressed adult for a mild first episode instead of a severe recurrent episode with psychotic features, but will barely know how to proceed with an adult diagnosed with a nonspecific mental disorder. Identifying a specific disorder improves communication with other clinicians, while also indicating to patients (and their caregivers, when available) the diagnostic acumen of the referring clinician. Diagnosis is, itself, a response to a patient's suffering, because giving a specific name to the seemingly unnamable is salutary. (It also improves communication with regulators and third-party payers, who frequently reimburse better for more specific diagnoses.)

Sometimes a specific diagnosis is inappropriate. When a clinician is uncertain or needs additional information, a provisional diagnosis is always preferable to a specific but inaccurate one. Just remember to eventually arrive at the most specific diagnosis possible. It is discouraging to review medical records in which a person's diagnosis remains poorly characterized for years.

Even if your diagnoses lack specificity, you can make them comprehensive. They should include all problems that are currently diminishing a person's ability to function: illnesses, general medical conditions, and psychosocial problems.

- To describe mental illnesses, use DSM-5-TR, including the adverse effects from psychiatric treatment that are described in Section II of DSM-5-TR.
- To describe general medical conditions, include those that currently affect a person's functioning while omitting well-healed injuries and resolved ailments.
- To describe psychosocial problems that influence a person's health, use the standardized list of ICD-11 Z codes. Several of the most relevant Z codes are found in Chapter 6 of this book, but the complete list of Z codes, numbered 00–99, are found in the ICD chapter called "Factors Influencing Health Status and Contact With Health Services," which can be found online at https://icd.who.int/browse11/l-m/en.

Finally, problems should be ordered hierarchically. The problems that are the focus of treatment should lead the list. For example, an older man may have hypertension, but if you are treating him for an episode of major depressive disorder following an intentional overdose, then his first two problems are his major depressive disorder and his suicide attempt. If you evaluate him again 2 months later and he has recovered from his depression and his ingestion, then his depressive episode and suicide attempt would be lower on the problem list. A well-ordered problem list communicates the focus of treatment to everyone who reads the record.

Patient and Caregiver Goals

A clinician develops the goals of treatment in conversation with their patient and, when appropriate and available, their caregivers. Sometimes practitioners ask about goals toward the end of a clinical conversation, but it is ideal to ask about treatment goals from the beginning, and then again throughout a conversation and treatment course. Checking in about treatment goals and progress toward achieving them is another way to establish a therapeutic alliance, the mutual commitment a clinician and a patient make to improve the patient's well-being.

The clinician and the patient establish the alliance when a patient identifies treatment goals and the clinician allies themselves with the patient in pursuit of those goals. By doing this early in the encounter, the clinician invariably increases the amount and reliability of information a patient offers.

More profoundly, the clinician helps motivate a patient's desire to change. So it helps to ask, often very directly, *"What is your treatment goal?"* Then, as the encounter progresses, frequently check in about additional goals, saying something like, *"I hear that you are concerned; should we address that as a treatment goal?"* By continuing to ask about treatment goals, a clinician clarifies the focus of treatment and further builds the alliance with a patient.

By the end of a conversation in which a clinician has frequently asked about treatment goals, it is usually straightforward to summarize the most pressing treatment goals. Do so by saying something like, *"It sounds like we have identified the most important treatment goals, but I want to be certain. Have we identified the right goals?"* These kinds of conversations ensure that a clinician's treatment goals will reflect a patient's desires, which usually increases their interest in pursuing the treatment plans. When possible and appropriate, phrase the treatment goals using the patient's own words.

Part of the challenge of working with persons with mental distress is bringing patients and caregivers together in pursuit of common goals. With patients, a clinician should identify goals early in an encounter. With caregivers, it helps to understand the relationship between a caregiver and a patient before asking about treatment goals. Different caregivers will be invested in a patient in different ways. Is the caregiver a spouse, sibling, child, parent, neighbor, religious authority, guardian, or home health aide? These relationships affect the treatment goals a caregiver identifies and their ability to meet those goals. A clinician needs to know how and why a caregiver is involved in a person's life when soliciting a caregiver's treatment goals.

Once the patient, caregiver (if available), and the clinician agree on treatment goals, it helps to consider the settings in which the goals will be pursued. If the problems you mutually identify occur mostly at home, then the goals should focus on the home. If the problems occur mostly at a facility like a school or nursing home, then your goals need to engage the facility's staff and other clients. If a clinician is seeing the patient in a primary care clinic, the treatment goal may include learning coping skills, developing new habits, or establishing care with a mental health clinician. If a clinician is seeing the patient in a hospital, the treatment goals usually address acute concerns, like decreasing suicidality or increasing mood.

Well-designed treatment goals help the clinician and patient feel a sense of accomplishment. Setting up realistic, achievable goals requires buy-in from the patient and caregiver that this is a goal they want to achieve and in which they find personal emotional value. The clinician should also consider the patient's age, functional ability, and physical or psychological characteristics, and set realistic expectations about what can be achieved in what timespan. The treatment goals a clinician sets with a patient should also be measurable, so they can know when the patient is, or is not, achieving the goals they have agreed upon, and should include a time frame in which they will be completed. For example, instead of telling a patient to "be more physically active," a clinician should set a specific, personal, and measurable goal for a designated time period such as: "Take your dog for a 10-minute walk three times a day for the next three months" and then have a patient keep a journal to keep track of their success rate. Sequential ways to develop an initial treatment plan are outlined below.

Sequential ways to develop an initial treatment plan

Step

1   Identify a patient's initial treatment goal.

2   Develop a therapeutic alliance with the patient.

3   Reach the most specific DSM-5-TR diagnosis for the patient.

4   Write a hierarchical, current problem list.

5   Rewrite the problem list into treatment goals.

6   Identify measurable and achievable goals from the available evidence base.

Step	
7	Customize the treatment for a patient's cultural background and available resources.
8	Assign responsibility for each goal to a member of the patient's treatment teams.
9	Monitor the progress toward each goal.
10	Revise the goals as a patient's situation changes.

Best Practices

One way to identify achievable and measurable goals is to personalize treatment goals to what has been shown in the medical literature to be possible to achieve. There are a number of strong texts to guide treatment planning (e.g., Reichenberg and Seligman 2016). Clinical practice guidelines can often inform a treatment plan. The American Psychiatric Association maintains a set of clinical practice guidelines, which may be found online at http://psychiatryonline.org/guidelines.

Chapter 11

The American Board of Psychiatry and Neurology Clinical Skills Evaluation

Board certification signals a physician's acquisition of the core skills of a competent practitioner. A psychiatrist's core skill is listening well in pursuit of understanding another person. To achieve board certification as a psychiatrist, a physician must thrice demonstrate their ability to interview and present a patient to an evaluating psychiatrist with the same skill as a competent practicing psychiatrist.

The American Board of Psychiatry and Neurology (ABPN) requires that an applicant demonstrate their skills by passing clinical skills evaluations (CSEs) with three separate patients. Each patient must be an actual rather than standardized patient. Each patient must be unknown to the applicant, though an applicant may receive a brief intake form about the patient. A non–English speaking patient may be interviewed during a CSE if the applicant and evaluator both speak the patient's language, but the patient's case must be presented in English.

Each CSE includes at least 30 minutes to interview a patient and 10–15 minutes to present the case, but training programs can provide supplementary time. Some training programs increase the time to simultaneously assess additional competencies.

In published surveys, most residents report positive experiences of the CSE (Rao et al. 2012).

Evaluations occur in the continuous presence of an evaluating psychiatrist who is currently certified by ABPN. The evaluating psychiatrist evaluates an applicant's ability to perform each of three skills—form a physician-patient relationship, conduct a psychiatric interview with a mental status examination, and present the resulting clinical case—at the level of a competent psychiatrist.

Evaluators assess an applicant's clinical skills using a standardized form measuring each of the three skills; the ABPN provides two standardized forms, Psych CSV v1 and Psych CSV v2, as fillable pdfs. On these forms, evaluators rate a resident's ability to perform each skill, and its constituent skills, on a scale from 1 to 8, with scores from 1 to 4 being unacceptable and scores from 5 to 8 being acceptable. For an examinee to pass the examination, a faculty member must score the resident at 5 or above on each skill. Alternately, residencies may develop their own forms and, with ABPN approval, employ them during evaluations. Additional information is available online at www.abpn.com.

The ABPN requires that the program director of an Accreditation Council for Graduate Medical Education (ACGME)–accredited psychiatry residency attest to the completion of three CSEs. Indeed, the ACGME requires at least an annual CSE—with added requirements for a formulation, differential diagnosis, and initial treatment plan—of each psychiatry trainee. An applicant can be examined at any point in their training; surveys suggest that the majority of applicants have their first evaluation during their first year of residency and complete the requirement during their third year of training (Juul et al. 2015). A program director attests for their own program's residents but may additionally attest for graduates of other psychiatry residencies.

While each residency training program creates its own rules for evaluations, every residency can learn from the counsel of peer programs. An ABPN task force of experienced psychiatric educators previously made several recommendations about how a CSE can enhance clinical training. The task force counseled selecting patients from a variety of the program's usual clinical settings so that applicants examine patients who accurately represent the people with mental illness found in treatment settings. They suggested allowing applicants an amount of interview time appropriate for the type of patient encounters, typically 30–45 minutes in acute settings and 45–60 minutes in other settings. The task force recommended using each CSE as a formative encounter, advising faculty to offer specific feedback that is actionable and constructive after each CSE. To help the faculty do so, they suggested training faculty evaluators, providing observational aids, identifying and defining criteria for each evaluated skill, and providing regular feedback to faculty evaluators (Jibson et al. 2012).

In a subsequent survey of psychiatry residency program directors, most program directors reported using the CSE as a teaching tool for feedback. When applicants failed a CSE, few programs required remediation. Ultimately, most program directors believed the evaluations accurately measure an applicant's skill and report that most applicants passed within three or four evaluations (Juul et al. 2015). Some observers are concerned by these reported pass rates on an examination that varies between training programs and are raising concerns that residency programs are incentivized to pass their own trainees. These observers are calling for changes in the evaluation process (Balon et al. 2020).

The evaluations of training psychiatrists will surely continue to change, but just as surely, all psychiatrists will benefit from continuing to practice their core clinical skill: listening well in pursuit of understanding.

Applicants can make the most of these examinations by receiving them as an opportunity to form the habits of a psychiatrist while they practice a psychiatrist's skills. Before an examination, an applicant should read the ABPN's instructions, ask their training director for the program's CSE form, and familiarize themselves, when possible, with the clinical setting in which they will be evaluated.

Practice until these skills become habits. Chapter 3, "The 30-Minute Diagnostic Interview," is one way to practice. Garner enough information to make a formulation, diagnosis, and initial treatment plan so you can meet the higher bar set by the ACGME. Remember that the ultimate goal is to show how you relate to and understand a person presenting with mental distress, and keep in mind that the most important skill to demonstrate is your ability to form a therapeutic alliance. After all, forming alliances with the distressed and the ill is the core act of a psychiatrist (Kinghorn and Nussbaum 2021).

Chapter 12

Selected DSM-5-TR Assessment Measures

In addition to its categorical diagnoses, DSM-5-TR includes a number of assessment tools for measuring symptoms, severity, and functional states that cross diagnostic categories. These measures are useful for screening for mental disorders, characterizing the degree of functional impairment associated with a mental disorder, and prioritizing clinical concerns. Because I designed this book for the diagnostic interview, I include in this chapter only the tools most useful for the diagnostic interview. The full range of assessment measures relevant to DSM-5-TR, including those for diagnostic severity, can be found online at www.psychiatry.org/dsm5.

Cultural Formulation Interview

As discussed in Chapter 4 ("Personalizing Diagnoses Through Dimensions"), the Cultural Formulation Interview (CFI) is not a scored rating system, but rather a series of prompts to help you explore a person's understanding of illness and health. The CFI can be incorporated into a diagnostic examination when you want to personalize the diagnosis and build a therapeutic alliance. A clinician can use either a single portion (called a *domain*) of the CFI, or the complete interview. The complete CFI, which is in Section III of DSM-5-TR, includes additional questions that expand upon each domain. The CFI's authors encouraged its adaptation by individual clinicians, so I often use the following operationalized adaptation, divided into six themes. Just as in the rest of the book, the italicized portions are interview prompts.

Introduction: *I would like to understand the problems that bring you here so that I can help you more effectively. I want to know about your experience and ideas. I will ask some questions about what is go-*

ing on and how you are dealing with it. There are no right or wrong answers. I just want to know your views and those of other important people in your life.

Cultural definition of the problem: *What problems or concerns bring you to the clinic? What troubles you most about your problem? People often understand their problems in their own way, which may be similar to or different from how doctors explain the problem. How would you describe your problem to someone else? Sometimes people use particular words or phrases to talk about their problems. Is there a specific term or expression that describes your problem? If yes: What is it?*

Cultural perceptions of cause and context: *Why do you think this is happening to you? What do you think are the particular causes of your problem? Some people may explain their problem as the result of bad things that happen in their lives, problems with others, or a physical illness. Or they give a spiritual reason for, or identify some other cause of, their problem. Do you? What, if anything, makes your problem worse, or makes it harder to cope with? What have your family, friends, and other people in your life done that may have made your problem worse? What, if anything, makes your problem better, or helps you cope with it more easily?*

Role of cultural identity: *Is there anything about your background—for example, your culture, race, ethnicity, religion, or geographical origin—that is causing problems for you in your current life situation? If yes: In what way? On the other hand, is there anything about your background that helps you to cope with your current life situation? If yes: In what way?*

Cultural factors affecting self-coping and past help seeking: *Sometimes people consider various ways of making themselves feel better. What have you done on your own to cope with your problem? Often, people also look for help from other individuals, groups, or institutions to help them feel better. In the past, what kind of treatment or help from other sources have you sought for your problem? What type of help or treatment was most useful? How? What type of help or treatment was not useful? How? Has anything prevented you from getting the help you need—for example, cost or lack of insurance coverage, getting time off work or family responsibilities, concern about stigma or discrimination, or lack of services that understand your language or culture? If yes: What got in the way?*

Current help seeking: *Now let's talk about the help you would be getting here. Is there anything about my own background that might make it difficult for me to understand or help you with your problem?*

How can I and others at our facility be most helpful to you? What kind of help would you like from us now, as specialists in mental health?

Conclusion: Thank the person for participation, summarize the main findings, and transition back to the remainder of your interview.

World Health Organization Disability Assessment Schedule 2.0

The authors of DSM-5-TR adopted the World Health Organization Disability Assessment Schedule 2.0 (WHODAS 2.0) for assessing a person's function in six domains: cognition, mobility, self-care, getting along, life activities, and participation. WHODAS 2.0 is available in several versions: 12- and 36-question versions that can be self-administered, proxy-administered, or interviewer-administered (see World Health Organization 2010).

For a DSM-5-TR diagnostic interview, DSM-5-TR includes the 36-item self-administered version in Section III. WHODAS 2.0 includes background questions about, among other topics, age, gender, educational attainment, and marital and occupational status. You can obtain the WHODAS 2.0 online at www.who.int/classifications/icf/whodasii/en. However, while the WHODAS 2.0 is a validated, reliable instrument, it was not designed specifically for assessing persons with mental illness and should be supplemented by an interview evaluating a patient's housing, physical health, social relationships, and employment (Konecky et al. 2014).

Clinician-Rated Dimensions of Psychosis Symptom Severity

The authors of DSM-5-TR included the Clinician-Rated Dimensions of Psychosis Symptom Severity, an 8-item measure that may be completed by the clinician at the time of the clinical assessment for a patient with a psychotic disorder. Each item asks the clinician to rate the severity of each symptom as experienced by the individual during the past 7 days. The measure may be used at regular intervals to chart a patient's clinical progress.

Name: _____ Age: _____ Date: _____

Instructions: Based on all the information you have on the individual and using your clinical judgment, please rate (with checkmark) the presence and severity of the following symptoms as experienced by the individual, when each symptom was at its most severe, in the past seven (7) days.

Domain	0	1	2	3	4	Score
I. Hallucinations	☐ Not present	☐ Equivocal (severity or duration not sufficient to be considered psychosis)	☐ Present, but mild (little pressure to act upon voices, not very bothered by voices)	☐ Present and moderate (some pressure to respond to voices, or is somewhat bothered by voices)	☐ Present and severe (severe pressure to respond to voices, or is very bothered by voices)	
II. Delusions	☐ Not present	☐ Equivocal (severity or duration not sufficient to be considered psychosis)	☐ Present, but mild (little pressure to act upon delusional beliefs, not very bothered by beliefs)	☐ Present and moderate (some pressure to act upon beliefs, or is somewhat bothered by beliefs)	☐ Present and severe (severe pressure to act upon beliefs, or is very bothered by beliefs)	
III. Disorganized speech	☐ Not present	☐ Equivocal (severity or duration not sufficient to be considered disorganization)	☐ Present, but mild (some difficulty following speech)	☐ Present and moderate (speech often difficult to follow)	☐ Present and severe (speech almost impossible to follow)	

Domain	0	1	2	3	4	Score
IV. Abnormal psychomotor behavior	☐ Not present	☐ Equivocal (severity or duration not sufficient to be considered abnormal psychomotor behavior)	☐ Present, but mild (occasional abnormal or bizarre motor behavior or catatonia)	☐ Present and moderate (frequent abnormal or bizarre motor behavior or catatonia)	☐ Present and severe (abnormal or bizarre motor behavior or catatonia almost constant)	
V. Negative symptoms (restricted emotional expression or avolition)	☐ Not present	☐ Equivocal decrease in facial expressivity, prosody, gestures, or self-initiated behavior	☐ Present, but mild decrease in facial expressivity, prosody, gestures, or self-initiated behavior	☐ Present and moderate decrease in facial expressivity, prosody, gestures, or self-initiated behavior	☐ Present and severe decrease in facial expressivity, prosody, gestures, or self-initiated behavior	
VI. Impaired cognition	☐ Not present	☐ Equivocal (cognitive function not clearly outside the range expected for age or SES; i.e., within 0.5 SD of mean)	☐ Present, but mild (some reduction in cognitive function; below expected for age and SES, 0.5–1 SD from mean)	☐ Present and moderate (clear reduction in cognitive function; below expected for age and SES, 1–2 SD from mean)	☐ Present and severe (severe reduction in cognitive function; below expected for age and SES, > 2 SD from mean)	

Domain	0	1	2	3	4	Score
VII. Depression	☐ Not present	☐ Equivocal (occasionally feels sad, down, depressed, or hopeless; concerned about having failed someone or at something but not preoccupied)	☐ Present, but mild (frequent periods of feeling very sad, down, moderately depressed, or hopeless; concerned about having failed someone or at something, with some preoccupation)	☐ Present and moderate (frequent periods of deep depression or hopelessness; preoccupation with guilt, having done wrong)	☐ Present and severe (deeply depressed or hopeless daily; delusional guilt or unreasonable self-reproach grossly out of proportion to circumstances)	
VIII. Mania	☐ Not present	☐ Equivocal (occasional elevated, expansive, or irritable mood or some restlessness)	☐ Present, but mild (frequent periods of somewhat elevated, expansive, or irritable mood or restlessness)	☐ Present and moderate (frequent periods of extensively elevated, expansive, or irritable mood or restlessness)	☐ Present and severe (daily and extensively elevated, expansive, or irritable mood or restlessness)	

Note. SD = standard deviation; SES = socioeconomic status.

Chapter 13

Dimensional Diagnosis of Personality Disorders

DSM-5-TR includes two distinct methods for diagnosing personality traits and disorders. The first method is a *categorical* method. This categorical method is included in the main section of DSM-5-TR for clinical use and is incorporated into the diagnostic interview in Chapters 3 ("The 30-Minute Diagnostic Interview") and 6 ("The DSM-5-TR Diagnostic Interview") of this guide. However, the second method is a *dimensional* method that will be novel for most interviewers. At present, the dimensional model is recommended for the use of researchers but is included in Section III of DSM-5-TR as an emerging model that may eventually replace the more-familiar categorical model, and it is useful today for all clinicians and patients.

The dimensional model of personality disorders requires an introduction because it initially appears clinically unwieldy (e.g. Skodol et al. 2015; Weekers et al. 2020).

One way to understand this is to consider the cluster model. When personality disorders are organized into Clusters A, B, and C, they are being classed along personality spectra: odd-eccentric, dramatic-emotional, and anxious-fearful. However, the cluster model is dimensional only between diagnoses.

A fully dimensional model needs to reckon with how personality traits occur across and outside disorders. For example, to allow a clinician to observe the submissive traits in one patient whose presentation meets criteria for borderline personality disorder while recording the same traits in another patient whose presentation meets the criteria for avoidant personality disorder, and do so without diagnosing separate personality disorders. Doing so allows several of the personality disorders in the categorical model to be unnecessary in the dimensional model. The dimensional model also allows you to go beyond determining if a person does (or does not) have a personality disorder, to assess the extent to which a personality disorder is associated with functional impairment in their relationships with other people and their sense of self. In short, if the disadvantage of the dimensional model is our lack of familiarity, its advantage is that it allows us to produce more sophisticated accounts of a person's character structure.

In this chapter, I include three tools to introduce the dimensional model of personality disorders. The first, the Level of Personality Functioning Scale, is also found in Section III of DSM-5-TR. The scale allows you to assess the level of functional impairment associated with the personality traits or disorders you diagnose. The second, the Personality Trait Rating Form, is also found in Section III of DSM-5-TR. This form allows you to observe the presence and severity of the 25 traits that underlie personality disorders. The third, a diagnostic interview, draws on the proposed dimensional diagnostic criteria for personality disorders in Section III of DSM-5-TR. As in the other sections of this pocket guide, it begins with a screening question and is followed by subsequent questions to determine a specific diagnosis.

Level of Personality Functioning Scale

For each person you evaluate, DSM-5-TR advises evaluation of their personality traits in relation to their ability to function both personally and interpersonally. This evaluation can guide treatment planning and influence prognosis, as discussed in Chapter 4, "Personalizing Diagnoses Through Dimensions."

In order to use it, you need sufficient clinical and historical information to differentiate five levels of functioning impairment, ranging from *little or no impairment* (Level 0) to *extreme impairment* (Level 4).

Using the following descriptions as your guide, indicate the level that most closely characterizes a patient's self-functioning and interpersonal functioning.

Level	Self		Interpersonal	
	Identity	Self-Direction	Empathy	Intimacy
0 (Little or no impairment)	• Ongoing awareness of a unique self; maintains role-appropriate boundaries. • Consistent and self-regulated positive self-esteem, with accurate self-appraisal. • Capable of experiencing, tolerating, and regulating a full range of emotions.	• Sets and aspires to reasonable goals based on a realistic assessment of personal capacities. • Utilizes appropriate standards of behavior, attaining fulfillment in multiple realms. • Can reflect on, and make constructive meaning of, internal experience.	• Capable of accurately understanding others' experiences and motivations in most situations. • Comprehends and appreciates others' perspectives, even if disagreeing. • Is aware of the effect of own actions on others.	• Maintains multiple satisfying and enduring relationships in personal and community life. • Desires and engages in a number of caring, close, and reciprocal relationships. • Strives for cooperation and mutual benefit and flexibly responds to a range of others' ideas, emotions, and behaviors.

Level	Self		Interpersonal	
	Identity	Self-Direction	Empathy	Intimacy
1 (Some impairment)	• Relatively intact sense of self, with some decrease in clarity of boundaries when strong emotions and mental distress are experienced. • Self-esteem diminished at times, with overly critical or somewhat distorted self-appraisal. • Strong emotions may be distressing, associated with a restriction in range of emotional experience.	• Excessively goal-directed, somewhat goal-inhibited, or conflicted about goals. • May have an unrealistic or socially inappropriate set of personal standards, limiting some aspects of fulfillment. • Able to reflect on internal experiences, but may overemphasize a single (e.g., intellectual, emotional) type of self-knowledge.	• Somewhat compromised in ability to appreciate and understand others' experiences; may tend to see others as having unreasonable expectations or a wish for control. • Although capable of considering and understanding different perspectives, resists doing so. • Inconsistent in awareness of effect of own behavior on others.	• Able to establish enduring relationships in personal and community life, with some limitations on degree of depth and satisfaction. • Capacity and desire to form intimate and reciprocal relationships, but may be inhibited in meaningful expression and sometimes constrained if intense emotions or conflicts arise. • Cooperation may be inhibited by unrealistic standards; somewhat limited in ability to respect or respond to others' ideas, emotions, and behaviors.

| Level | Self | | Interpersonal | |
	Identity	Self-Direction	Empathy	Intimacy
2 (Moderate impairment)	• Excessive dependence on others for identity definition, with compromised boundary delineation. • Vulnerable self-esteem controlled by exaggerated concern about external evaluation, with a wish for approval. Sense of incompleteness or inferiority, with compensatory inflated, or deflated, self-appraisal. • Emotional regulation depends on positive external appraisal. Threats to self-esteem may engender strong emotions such as rage or shame.	• Goals are more often a means of gaining external approval than self-generated, and thus may lack coherence and/or stability. • Personal standards may be unreasonably high (e.g., a need to be special or please others) or low (e.g., not consonant with prevailing social values). Fulfillment is compromised by a sense of lack of authenticity. • Impaired capacity to reflect upon internal experience.	• Hyperattuned to the experience of others, but only with respect to perceived relevance to self. • Excessively self-referential; significantly compromised ability to appreciate and understand others' experiences and to consider alternative perspectives. • Generally unaware of or unconcerned about effect of own behavior on others, or unrealistic appraisal of own effect.	• Capacity and desire to form relationships in personal and community life, but connections may be largely superficial. • Intimate relationships are largely based on meeting self-regulatory and self-esteem needs, with an unrealistic expectation of being perfectly understood by others. • Tends not to view relationships in reciprocal terms, and cooperates predominantly for personal gain.

Level	Self		Interpersonal	
	Identity	**Self-Direction**	**Empathy**	**Intimacy**
3 (Severe impairment)	• A weak sense of autonomy/agency; experience of a lack of identity, or emptiness. Boundary definition is poor or rigid: may be overidentification with others, overemphasis on independence from others, or vacillation between these. • Fragile self-esteem is easily influenced by events, and self-image lacks coherence. Self-appraisal is unnuanced: self-loathing, self-aggrandizing, or an illogical, unrealistic combination. • Emotions may be rapidly shifting or a chronic, unwavering feeling of despair.	• Difficulty establishing and/or achieving personal goals. • Internal standards for behavior are unclear or contradictory. Life is experienced as meaningless or dangerous. • Significantly compromised ability to reflect upon and understand own mental processes.	• Ability to consider and understand the thoughts, feelings, and behavior of other people is significantly limited; may discern very specific aspects of others' experience, particularly vulnerabilities and suffering. • Generally unable to consider alternative perspectives; highly threatened by differences of opinion or alternative viewpoints. • Confusion or unawareness of impact of own actions on others; often bewildered about people's thoughts and actions, with destructive motivations frequently misattributed to others.	• Some desire to form relationships in community and personal life is present, but capacity for positive and enduring connection is significantly impaired. • Relationships are based on a strong belief in the absolute need for the intimate other(s), and/or expectations of abandonment or abuse. Feelings about intimate involvement with others alternate between fear/rejection and desperate desire for connection. • Little mutuality: others are conceptualized primarily in terms of how they affect the self (negatively or positively); cooperative efforts are often disrupted due to the perception of slights from others.

Level	Self		Interpersonal	
	Identity	Self-Direction	Empathy	Intimacy
4 (Extreme impairment)	• Experience of a unique self and sense of agency/autonomy are virtually absent, or are organized around perceived external persecution. Boundaries with others are confused or lacking. • Weak or distorted self-image easily threatened by interactions with others; significant distortions and confusion around self-appraisal. • Emotions not congruent with context or internal experience. Hatred and aggression may be dominant affects, although they may be disavowed and attributed to others.	• Poor differentiation of thoughts from actions, so goal-setting ability is severely compromised, with unrealistic or incoherent goals. • Internal standards for behavior are virtually lacking. Genuine fulfillment is virtually inconceivable. • Profound inability to constructively reflect upon own experience. Personal motivations may be unrecognized and/or experienced as external to self.	• Pronounced inability to consider and understand others' experience and motivation. • Attention to others' perspectives virtually absent (attention is hypervigilant, focused on need fulfillment and harm avoidance). • Social interactions can be confusing and disorienting.	• Desire for affiliation is limited because of profound disinterest or expectation of harm. Engagement with others is detached, disorganized, or consistently negative. • Relationships are conceptualized almost exclusively in terms of their ability to provide comfort or inflict pain and suffering. • Social/interpersonal behavior is not reciprocal; rather, it seeks fulfillment of basic needs or escape from pain.

Personality Trait Rating Form

It is sometimes clinically useful to create a detailed portrait of a person's personality traits. In the dimensional DSM-5-TR model for personality disorders, this is done by rating domains and facets of a person's usual personality—what they have been for the majority of the person's adult life. For each domain and facet, you rate how well the description assesses the person before you on this 4-point scale:

0	1	2	3
Very little or not at all descriptive	Mildly descriptive	Moderately descriptive	Extremely descriptive

Rating	Negative affectivity	Experiences negative emotions frequently and intensely

NOTE: Restricted Affectivity is listed under the Detachment heading, but the absence of this facet trait—i.e., a tendency to have strong reactions to emotionally arousing situations—should also be evaluated in rating the overall Negative Affectivity domain.

Emotional lability		Unstable emotional experiences and frequent mood changes; emotions that are easily aroused, intense, and/or out of proportion to events and circumstances
Anxiousness		Intense feelings of nervousness, tenseness, or panic in reaction to diverse situations; worry about the negative effects of past unpleasant experiences and future negative possibilities; feeling fearful, apprehensive, or threatened by uncertainty; fears of falling apart, losing control, or embarrassment
Separation insecurity		Fears of rejection by—and/or separation from—significant others, associated with fears of excessive dependency and complete loss of autonomy
Perseveration		Persistence at tasks long after the behavior has ceased to be functional or effective; continuance of the same behavior despite repeated failures
Submissiveness		Adaptation of one's behavior to the interests and desires of others
Hostility		Persistent or frequent angry feelings; anger or irritability in response to minor slights and insults; mean, nasty, or vengeful behavior
Depressivity		Frequent feelings of being down, miserable, and/or hopeless; difficulty recovering from such moods; pessimism about the future; pervasive shame; feelings of inferior self-worth; thoughts of suicide and suicidal behavior
Suspiciousness		Expectations of—and heightened sensitivity to—signs of interpersonal ill-intent or harm; doubts about loyalty and fidelity of others; feelings of persecution

Dimensional Diagnosis of Personality Disorders **239**

Rating	Detachment	Withdrawal from other people and from social interactions

NOTE: Because they are rated earlier, as part of Negative Affectivity, Depressivity and Suspiciousness are not listed again under the Detachment heading, but they should be evaluated in rating the overall Detachment domain.

Restricted affectivity	Little reaction to emotionally arousing situations; constricted emotional experience and expression; indifference or coldness
Withdrawal	Preference for being alone to being with others; reticence in social situations; avoidance of social contacts and activity; lack of initiation of social contact
Anhedonia	Lack of enjoyment from, engagement in, or energy for life's experiences; deficits in the capacity to feel pleasure or take interest in things
Intimacy avoidance	Avoidance of close or romantic relationships, interpersonal attachments, and intimate sexual relationships

Rating	Antagonism	Engaging in behaviors that put the person at odds with other people

NOTE: Because it is rated earlier, as part of Negative Affectivity, Hostility is not listed again under the Antagonism heading, but it should be evaluated in rating the overall Antagonism domain.

Manipulativeness	Frequent use of subterfuge to influence or control others; use of seduction, charm, glibness, or ingratiation to achieve one's ends
Deceitfulness	Dishonesty and fraudulence; misrepresentation of self; embellishment or fabrication when relating events
Grandiosity	Feelings of entitlement, either overt or covert; self-centeredness; firmly holding to the belief that one is better than others; condescending toward others
Attention seeking	Excessive attempts to attract and be the focus of the attention of others; admiration seeking
Callousness	Lack of concern for feelings or problems of others; lack of guilt or remorse about the negative or harmful effects of one's actions on others; aggression; sadism

Rating	Disinhibition/ compulsivity	Engaging in behaviors on impulse, without reflecting on potential future consequences

NOTE: Compulsivity is the opposite of disinhibition and, if present, should be recorded at the facet level as Rigid Perfectionism in the absence of other disinhibition facets. Rigid Perfectionism reflects Compulsivity, which is the opposite of disinhibition and is therefore located in the Disinhibition domain. If present, Compulsivity should be recorded at the facet level as a higher Rigid Perfectionism score accompanied by lower scores on other disinhibition facets.

Irresponsibility	Disregard for—and failure to honor—financial and other obligations or commitments; lack of respect for—and lack of follow-through on—agreements and promises
Impulsivity	Acting on the spur of the moment in response to immediate stimuli; acting on a momentary basis without a plan or consideration of outcomes; difficulty establishing and following plans; a sense of urgency and self-harming behavior under emotional distress
Distractibility	Difficulty concentrating and focusing on tasks; attention is easily diverted by extraneous stimuli; difficulty maintaining goal-focused behavior
Risk taking	Engagement in dangerous, risky, and potentially self-damaging activities, unnecessarily and without regard to consequences; boredom proneness and thoughtless initiation of activities to counter boredom; lack of concern for one's limitations and denial of the reality of personal danger
(lack of) Rigid perfectionism	Rigid insistence on everything being flawless, perfect, without errors or faults, including one's own and others' performance; sacrificing of timeliness to ensure correctness in every detail; believing that there is only one right way to do things; difficulty changing ideas and/or viewpoint; preoccupation with details, organization, and order

Rating	Psychoticism	Unusual and bizarre experiences
	Unusual beliefs and experiences	Thought content that is viewed by others as bizarre or idiosyncratic; unusual experiences of reality
	Eccentricity	Odd, unusual, or bizarre behavior or appearance; saying unusual or inappropriate things
	Cognitive and perceptual dysregulation	Odd or unusual thought processes; vague, circumstantial, metaphorical, overelaborate, or stereotyped thought or speech; odd experiences in various sensory modalities

DSM-5-TR, pp. 881–901

Screening questions: *When you look over your life, does it seem like your basic sense of who you are, your ability to accurately estimate the quality of your own life, and your ability to experience and regulate emotions have been unstable or have changed frequently? When you look over your life, does it seem like you struggled to consistently and purposefully pursue both short- and long-term goals for yourself?*

If yes to either question, ask: *When you look over your life, does it seem like you repeatedly struggle to appreciate the experiences of other people, to tolerate different perspectives, and to understand the effect of your behavior on other people? Do you really struggle to make and maintain deep positive connections with other people?*

If yes to either question, ask: *When people look over their lives, they can often identify persistent habits or traits that recur throughout their lives. When you look over your life, can you see that one of these traits is relatively stable over time: having a negative sense of yourself that changes quickly in response to circumstances; a compulsive focus on getting things perfect or rightly ordered; avoiding or withdrawing from emotional intimate relationships to the extent that you feel detached from other people; a commitment to behaviors and beliefs that many other people consider unusual or eccentric; a persistent sense that you are much more accomplished or deserving than other people; or a pattern of behaviors that many other people have found manipulative, deceitful, hostile, or irresponsible?*

- If negative affectivity as characterized by an unstable negative mood predominates, proceed to borderline personality disorder criteria.

- If compulsivity predominates, proceed to obsessive-compulsive personality disorder criteria.
- If detachment predominates, proceed to avoidant personality disorder criteria.
- If psychoticism characterized by unusual or eccentric behaviors predominates, proceed to schizotypal personality disorder criteria.
- If antagonism characterized by manipulativeness, deceitfulness, hostility, and irresponsibility predominates, proceed to antisocial (dissocial) personality disorder criteria.
- If antagonism characterized by grandiosity and attention seeking predominates, proceed to narcissistic personality disorder criteria.

1. Borderline Personality Disorder

    a. Inclusion: Requires impairments in self-functioning as manifested by at least <u>one</u> of the following difficulties.

        i. Identity: *Do you have a very unstable or poorly developed sense of who you are? Are you excessively critical of yourself? Do you chronically feel empty? At times of stress, do you ever feel like you are an outside observer of your mind, thoughts, feelings, sensations, body, or your whole self or experience people or places as unreal, dreamlike, foggy, lifeless, or visually distorted?*

        ii. Self-direction: *Are your aspirations, career plans, goals, and values unstable and frequently changing?*

    b. Inclusion: Also requires impairment in interpersonal functioning as manifested by at least <u>one</u> of the following difficulties.

        i. Empathy: *Do you struggle to recognize the needs and feelings of other people? Are you prone to feeling slighted or insulted? When you think about other people, do you think mostly about their negative qualities or their weaknesses?*

        ii. Intimacy: *Do you worry that if people get close to you, they will abandon you? Are most of your close relationships intense and unstable? Do you alternate between feeling as though the people in your life are really good and really bad? Do you alternate between being really involved with other people and then withdrawing from relationships?*

    c. Inclusion: Also requires pathological personality traits from at least <u>one</u> of the following domains.

i. Negative affectivity, characterized by at least <u>one</u> of the following:

- Emotional lability: *Are your emotions easily aroused or intense? Are your emotions often much stronger than the event or circumstance that triggered them?*
- Anxiousness: *Do you often have intense feelings of nervousness, tension, or panic, especially when stressed? Do you often feel afraid of uncertainty? Do you worry about how negative experiences in your past will affect your future? Do you fear falling apart or losing control?*
- Separation insecurity: *Do you really fear rejection by or separation from the people closest to you?*
- Depressivity: *Do you frequently feel down, miserable, or hopeless? Do you find it hard to recover from these moods? Are you very pessimistic about the future? Do you often feel ashamed of yourself or feel that you are worthless? Do you frequently think about harming or killing yourself?*

ii. Disinhibition, characterized by at least <u>one</u> of the following:

- Impulsivity: *Do you often act on the spur of the moment, without a plan or consideration for the outcome? Do you have difficulty establishing or following plans? When you are stressed, do you feel a sense of urgency or a desire to harm yourself?*
- Risk taking: *Do you frequently engage in dangerous, risky, and potentially self-damaging activities without regard to their consequences?*

iii. Antagonism, characterized by the following:

- Hostility: *Are you frequently angry or irritable, especially in response to minor slights and insults?*

d. Exclusions

i. If the impairments in personality functioning and the expression of personality traits are unstable over time and inconsistent across situations, do not make the diagnosis.

ii. If the impairments in personality functioning and the personality trait expressions are normative for a person's developmental stage or sociocultural environment, do not make the diagnosis.

iii. If the impairments in personality functioning and the personality trait expressions are solely attributable to the physiological effects of another medical condition or a substance, do not make the diagnosis.

e. Modifiers

    i. Descriptive features

- More pervasive negative affectivity
- More pervasive detachment
- More pervasive antagonism
- More pervasive disinhibition
- More pervasive psychoticism
- Level of personality functioning (0–4) (see Level of Personality Functioning Scale on pp. 232–237 in this chapter)

    ii. Course

- In remission

f. Alternative: If a person exhibits significant impairment in self and interpersonal functioning but does not meet criteria for a specific personality disorder, consider personality disorder—trait specified (full proposed criteria are in DSM-5-TR, p. 890). This diagnosis allows you to specify the domains in which pathological personality domains—negative affectivity, detachment, antagonism, disinhibition, and psychoticism—are present and to diagnose the disorder. If you desire, you can use the specific trait facets within each domain to particularize the diagnosis. (You can see a list of these facets in the Personality Trait Rating Form on pp. 238–242 of this chapter.)

2. Obsessive-Compulsive Personality Disorder

a. Inclusion: Requires impairments in self-functioning as manifested by at least <u>one</u> of the following difficulties.

    i. Identity: *Do you find that your sense of who you are and what makes you valuable as a person comes mostly from your work or how productive you are? Is it so difficult for you to experience and express strong emotions that it would be fair to characterize your ability to do so as constricted?*

    ii. Self-direction: *Do you have such a strong need to do your work or duty well and thoroughly that you find it difficult to complete tasks? Do you aspire to moral standards that are so high that it is difficult for you to realize goals?*

b. Inclusion: Also requires impairment in interpersonal functioning as manifested by at least <u>one</u> of the following difficulties.

   i. Empathy: *Do you struggle to understand and appreciate the ideas, feelings, or behaviors of other people?*

   ii. Intimacy: *In comparison to your work life, do you usually perceive relationships as secondary, or a lower priority? Does your need to be right or to not change your position frequently make it difficult to make and maintain relationships with other people?*

c. Inclusion: Also requires pathological personality traits from <u>both</u> of the following domains.

   i. Compulsivity, characterized by the following:

      • Rigid perfectionism: *Do you usually insist on things in your life being flawless, perfect, or without errors or fault? Do you frequently sacrifice finishing an activity or project on time in order to make sure every detail is correct? Do you usually believe there is only one right way to do things? Do you have a difficult time altering your ideas or viewpoint, even when you become aware of a compelling alternative? Are you preoccupied with details, organization, and order?*

   ii. Negative affectivity, characterized by the following:

      • Perseveration: *Do you frequently continue working on a task long after doing so is no longer effective? Do you frequently continue the same behaviors even after they have repeatedly resulted in failure?*

d. Exclusions

   i. If the impairments in personality functioning and the expression of personality traits are unstable over time and inconsistent across situations, do not make the diagnosis.

   ii. If the impairments in personality functioning and the personality trait expressions are normative for a person's developmental stage or sociocultural environment, do not make the diagnosis.

   iii. If the impairments in personality functioning and the personality trait expressions are solely attributable to the physiological effects of another medical condition or a substance, do not make the diagnosis.

    e. Modifiers

       i. Descriptive features

- More pervasive negative affectivity
- More pervasive detachment
- More pervasive antagonism
- More pervasive disinhibition
- More pervasive psychoticism
- Level of personality functioning (0–4) (see Level of Personality Functioning Scale on pp. 232–237 in this chapter)

    f. Alternative: If a person exhibits significant impairment in self and interpersonal functioning but does not meet criteria for a specific personality disorder, consider personality disorder—trait specified (full proposed criteria are in DSM-5-TR, p. 890). The diagnosis allows you to specify the domains in which pathological personality domains—negative affectivity, detachment, antagonism, disinhibition, and psychoticism—are present and to diagnose the disorder. If you desire, you can use the specific trait facets within each domain to particularize the diagnosis. (You can see a list of these facets in the Personality Trait Rating Form on pp. 238–242 of this chapter.)

3. Avoidant Personality Disorder

    a. Inclusion: Requires impairments in self-functioning as manifested by at least <u>one</u> of the following difficulties.

       i. Identity: *Do you have such low self-esteem that you usually perceive yourself as socially inept, unappealing, or inferior to other people? Do you frequently experience painful feelings of humiliation or inadequacy when you consider yourself?*

      ii. Self-direction: *Do you set such unrealistic standards for your behavior that it makes you reluctant to pursue your goals, take personal risks, or engage in new activities that would require you to interact with other people?*

    b. Inclusion: Also requires impairment in interpersonal functioning as manifested by at least <u>one</u> of the following difficulties.

i. Empathy: *Do you frequently find that your thoughts are dominated by the possibility that other people will criticize or reject you?*

ii. Intimacy: *Are you usually reluctant to become involved with other people unless you can be certain they will like you? Do you find it hard to make and maintain relationships because you fear being ridiculed or shamed?*

c. Inclusion: Also requires pathological personality traits from <u>all</u> of the following domains.

i. Detachment, characterized by at least <u>one</u> of the following:

- Withdrawal: *In social situations, are you usually reserved, often to the point of not communicating unless it is necessary? Do you avoid social activity? Do you rarely begin or initiate social contact?*
- Intimacy avoidance: *Do you usually avoid close or romantic relationships, interpersonal attachments, and intimate sexual relationships?*
- Anhedonia: *Do you find it hard to be engaged in, or have energy for, life experiences? Do you find it difficult to feel pleasure?*

ii. Negative affectivity, characterized by the following:

- Anxiousness: *Do you frequently experience intense feelings of nervousness, tension, or panic, often in reaction to social situations? Do you often worry about the negative effects of unpleasant experiences from your past and how they might affect your future? When you confront a situation that is uncertain or unsettled, do you often feel fearful, apprehensive, or threatened?*

d. Exclusions

i. If the impairments in personality functioning and the expression of personality traits are unstable over time and inconsistent across situations, do not make the diagnosis.

ii. If the impairments in personality functioning and the personality trait expressions are normative for a person's developmental stage or sociocultural environment, do not make the diagnosis.

iii. If the impairments in personality functioning and the personality trait expressions are solely attributable to the physiological effects of another medical condition or a substance, do not make the diagnosis.

e. Modifiers

   i. Descriptive features

- More pervasive negative affectivity
- More pervasive detachment
- More pervasive antagonism
- More pervasive disinhibition
- More pervasive psychoticism
- Level of personality functioning (0–4) (see Level of Personality Functioning Scale on pp. 232–237 in this chapter)

f. Alternative: If a person exhibits significant impairment in self-functioning and interpersonal functioning, but does not meet criteria for a specific personality disorder, consider personality disorder—trait specified (full criteria are in DSM-5-TR, p. 890). The diagnosis allows you to specify the domains in which pathological personality domains—negative affectivity, detachment, antagonism, disinhibition, and psychoticism—are present and to diagnose the disorder. If you desire, you can use the specific trait facets within each domain to particularize the diagnosis. (You can see a list of these facets in the Personality Trait Rating Form on pp. 238–242 of this chapter.)

4. Schizotypal Personality Disorder

a. Inclusion: Requires impairments in self-functioning as manifested by at least <u>one</u> of the following difficulties.

   i. Identity: *Do you often find yourself confused about the boundaries between yourself and other people? Do other people ever tell you that you seem indifferent or aloof?*

   ii. Self-direction: *Do you frequently find it difficult to make realistic or coherent goals?*

b. Inclusion: Also requires impairment in interpersonal functioning as manifested by at least <u>one</u> of the following difficulties.

   i. Empathy: *Do you often find it difficult to understand how your behaviors affect other people? Do you often find that you misunderstand other people's behaviors and motivations?*

ii. Intimacy: *Are you so anxious or distrustful of other people that you struggle to make close friendships or other relationships?*

c. Inclusion: Also requires pathological personality traits from at least <u>one</u> of the following domains.

i. Psychoticism, characterized by at least <u>one</u> of the following:

- Eccentricity: *Do other people often respond to you as if your behavior or appearance was odd or bizarre? Do other people often tell you that the things you say are inappropriate or unusual?*
- Cognitive and perceptual dysregulation: Odd or unusual thought processes; vague, circumstantial, metaphorical, overelaborate, or stereotyped thought or speech; odd sensations in various modalities. *Do other people often have trouble following your thought process? Do other people often struggle to understand your speech? Do you often experience odd sensations, like the feeling that something unnatural is on your skin or inside your body, or that you see or hear things other people cannot?*
- Unusual beliefs and experiences: *Do you sometimes have the sense that another person, whom other people cannot see, is present and speaking with you? Are you very superstitious? Are you preoccupied with paranormal or magical phenomena?*

ii. Detachment, characterized by at least <u>one</u> of the following:

- Restricted affectivity: *Do you notice that your emotional experiences and expressions stay within a narrow range and do not change much over time? Have other people told you that you do not respond to emotionally provocative situations as they expect? Have other people ever told you that you seem emotionally cold or indifferent?*
- Withdrawal: *Do you usually prefer to be alone? In social situations, are you usually reserved, often to the point of not communicating unless it is necessary? Do you avoid social activity? Do you rarely begin or initiate social contact?*

iii. Negative affectivity, characterized by the following:

- Suspiciousness: *Do you frequently doubt that other people will be faithful, loyal, and supportive of you? Do you often suspect that other people have negative or harmful intentions toward you? Do you often feel like other people are persecuting you?*

d. Exclusions

  i. If the impairments in personality functioning and the expression of personality traits are unstable over time and inconsistent across situations, do not make the diagnosis.
  ii. If the impairments in personality functioning and the personality trait expressions are normative for a person's developmental stage or sociocultural environment, do not make the diagnosis.
  iii. If the impairments in personality functioning and the personality trait expressions are solely attributable to the physiological effects of another medical condition or a substance, do not make the diagnosis.

e. Modifiers

  i. Descriptive features
     - More pervasive negative affectivity
     - More pervasive detachment
     - More pervasive antagonism
     - More pervasive disinhibition
     - More pervasive psychoticism
     - Level of personality functioning (0–4) (see Level of Personality Functioning Scale on pp. 232–237 in this chapter)

f. Alternative: If a person exhibits significant impairment in self and interpersonal functioning but does not meet criteria for a specific personality disorder, consider personality disorder—trait specified (full proposed criteria are in DSM-5-TR, p. 890). The diagnosis allows you to specify the domains in which pathological personality domains—negative affectivity, detachment, antagonism, disinhibition, and psychoticism—are present and to diagnose the disorder. If you desire, you can use the specific trait facets within each domain to particularize the diagnosis. (You can see a list of these facets in the Personality Trait Rating Form on pp. 238–242 of this chapter.)

5. Antisocial (Dissocial) Personality Disorder

   a. Inclusion: Requires impairments in self-functioning as manifested by at least <u>one</u> of the following difficulties.

      i. Identity: *When you think about what makes you feel proud of yourself, do you find that it is usually personal gain, pleasure, or the attainment and exercise of power? When you are making choices, do you usually think of how they will affect you more than how they will affect other people?*

      ii. Self-direction: *When you set short- and long-term goals, is your chief motivation to gratify your own needs and desires? How important is it to you that your goals follow commonly accepted rules and guidelines for what is ethical and legal?*

   b. Inclusion: Also requires impairment in interpersonal functioning as manifested by at least <u>one</u> of the following difficulties.

      i. Empathy: *How concerned are you about the feelings, needs, or suffering of other people? If you have ever hurt or mistreated someone else, did you feel remorse or regret after doing so?*

      ii. Intimacy: *Do you find that you are incapable of being in relationships with other people in which you are emotionally close and engaged? Have you often coerced, deceived, exploited, or intimidated other people in an effort to control them?*

   c. Inclusion: Also requires pathological personality traits from <u>all</u> of the following domains.

      i. Antagonism, characterized by at least <u>one</u> of the following:

         • Manipulativeness: *Do you frequently charm or seduce other people to achieve something you desire? Do you frequently deceive other people in order to influence or control them?*
         • Deceitfulness: *Do you often misrepresent yourself by claiming accomplishments or qualities that are not your own? Do you often embellish stories and make up events?*
         • Callousness: *When you hear about other people's feelings or problems, do you usually feel disinterested or unsympathetic? When you learn that your own ac-*

tions have harmed someone else, do you feel guilty afterward? Do you find it pleasurable to inflict pain and suffering on another person?

- Hostility: *Are you frequently or even always angry? When someone slights or insults you, does it often make you irritable or even aggressive? Are you often rude, nasty, or vengeful?*

ii. Disinhibition, characterized by at least <u>one</u> of the following:

- Irresponsibility: *When you enter into agreements or make promises, do you often disrespect and fail to follow through on your commitments? When you have familial, financial, and other obligations, do you often disregard and fail to honor them?*
- Impulsivity: *Do you often struggle to formulate and follow a plan? Do you often act on the spur of the moment, without a plan or consideration of the consequences?*
- Risk taking: *Do you often engage in dangerous, risky, and potentially self-damaging activities with little thought to the consequences? Are you easily bored, and do you often start activities without thinking as a way to counter your boredom?*

d. Exclusions

i. If the impairments in personality functioning and the expression of personality traits are unstable over time and inconsistent across situations, do not make the diagnosis.

ii. If the impairments in personality functioning and the personality trait expressions are normative for a person's developmental stage or sociocultural environment, do not make the diagnosis.

iii. If the impairments in personality functioning and the personality trait expressions are solely attributable to the physiological effects of another medical condition or a substance, do not make the diagnosis.

e. Modifiers

i. Descriptive features

- More pervasive negative affectivity
- More pervasive detachment

- More pervasive antagonism
- More pervasive disinhibition
- More pervasive psychoticism
- Level of personality functioning (0–4) (see Level of Personality Functioning Scale on pp. 232–237 in this chapter)

    ii. Specifiers

- With psychopathic features specifier: Use when a person exhibits a lack of anxiety or fear and a bold, efficacious interpersonal style. Psychopathy comparatively emphasizes affective and interpersonal characteristics over the behavioral components.

  f. Alternative: If a person exhibits significant impairment in self-functioning and interpersonal functioning but does not meet criteria for a specific personality disorder, consider personality disorder—trait specified (full proposed criteria are in DSM-5-TR, p. 890). The diagnosis allows you to specify the domains in which pathological personality domains—negative affectivity, detachment, antagonism, disinhibition, and psychoticism—are present and to diagnose the disorder. If you desire, you can use the specific trait facets within each domain to particularize the diagnosis. (You can see a list of these facets in the Personality Trait Rating Form on pp. 238–242 of this chapter.)

6. Narcissistic Personality Disorder

  a. Inclusion: Requires impairments in self-functioning as manifested by at least <u>one</u> of the following difficulties.

    i. Identity: *Do you define yourself mostly in relationship to other people? Does the pride you take in yourself depend on how other people perceive and respond to you? Do you find that your emotions fluctuate in response to your estimation of the quality of your life?*

    ii. Self-direction: *Do you find it hard to understand what motivates you to make decisions and set goals? Do you usually set goals for yourself based on how other people will perceive your goals? Do you set standards for yourself really high to reflect how exceptional you are? Alternatively, do you set standards for yourself really low to reflect that you are entitled to whatever you achieve?*

b. Inclusion: Also requires impairment in interpersonal functioning as manifested by at least <u>one</u> of the following difficulties.

  i. Empathy: *Are you very attuned to the reactions other people have to you? Do you frequently think about how you affect other people? Do you find it hard to recognize or identify with the feelings and needs of other people?*

  ii. Intimacy: *In your relationships with other people, do you find that you are interested in other people and their experiences in terms of what they mean to you and your life? Do most of your relationships stay casual or on the surface? Do you value relationships with other people as a way to maintain your self-esteem?*

c. Inclusion: Also requires pathological personality traits from this domain.

  i. Antagonism, characterized by <u>both</u> of the following:

   • Grandiosity: *Do you deserve or have a right to particular treatments because of your excellent personal qualities? Do you believe that you are better or superior to other people? Do you often act in a way that makes other people inferior to you?*

   • Attention seeking: *Do you really like being the center of attention? Do you find that you often seek and attract the attention or admiration of other people?*

d. Exclusions

  i. If the impairments in personality functioning and the expression of personality traits are unstable over time and inconsistent across situations, do not make the diagnosis.

  ii. If the impairments in personality functioning and the personality trait expressions are normative for a person's developmental stage or sociocultural environment, do not make the diagnosis.

  iii. If the impairments in personality functioning and the personality trait expressions are solely attributable to the physiological effects of another medical condition or a substance, do not make the diagnosis.

e. Modifiers
   i. Descriptive features
       • More pervasive negative affectivity
       • More pervasive detachment
       • More pervasive antagonism
       • More pervasive disinhibition
       • More pervasive psychoticism
       • Level of personality functioning (0–4)
         (see Level of Personality Functioning Scale
         on pp. 232–237 in this chapter)
f. Alternative: If a person exhibits significant impairment
    in self-functioning and interpersonal functioning but
    does not meet criteria for a specific personality disor-
    der, consider personality disorder—trait specified (full
    criteria are in DSM-5-TR, p. 890). The diagnosis allows
    you to specify the domains in which pathological per-
    sonality domains—negative affectivity, detachment,
    antagonism, disinhibition, and psychoticism—are pres-
    ent and to diagnose the disorder. If you desire, you can
    use the specific trait facets within each domain to par-
    ticularize the diagnosis. (You can see a list of these fac-
    ets in the Personality Trait Rating Form on pp. 238–242
    of this chapter.)

Chapter 14

Alternative Diagnostic Systems and Rating Scales

DSM-5-TR provides clinicians a common vocabulary for characterizing the mental distress they observe in patents. Other communities use alternative vocabularies when describing the experiences of a person experiencing mental distress or illness (cf. Clark et al. 2017).

Alternative Diagnostic Systems

Culture-Specific Diagnostic Systems

The experience of mental illness and distress are always mediated through culture, which structures the human experience of health, illness, and receiving care. DSM-5-TR renews attention to the roles culture plays in mental disorders, building upon the development of the Cultural Formulation Interview, which is included in Chapter 12, and can be explored extensively elsewhere (Lewis-Fernández et al. 2016). Outside of DSM-5-TR, culture-specific psychiatric diagnostic systems are used in particular countries and regions, including China (Chen 2002), Cuba (Otero-Ojeda 2002), Japan (Nakane and Nakane 2002), and Latin America (Berganza and Mezzich 2004), and can be seen in specific faith traditions like Islam (Keshavarzi et al. 2020).

International Classification of Diseases

Across cultures, the World Health Organization maintains its own descriptive diagnostic system, the International Statistical Classification of Diseases and Related Health Problems, commonly called just the International Classification of Diseases or "ICD." The current, eleventh revision, or ICD-11, includes mental disorders within a catalog of all medical diseases. While most clinicians outside the United States use ICD-11 to diagnose mental disorders, ICD-11 was primarily designed to help epidemiologists track the incidence and prevalence of disease for public health interventions, so it provides less information for each diagnosis than DSM-5-TR. Despite their different designs, DSM-5-TR and ICD-11 essentially assign the same codes to psychiatric diagnoses, and these shared codes are widely used by insurers and regulators. The sixth chapter of ICD-11, "Mental, Behavioural or Neurodevelopmental Disorders," includes most of the diagnoses relevant for a diagnostic interview. However, sleep-wake disorders, sexual dysfunctions, and gender incongruence are coded in other chapters of ICD-11. Some clinicians may prefer ICD-11 because it is freely available online, commonly used by electronic health records, provides diagnostic guidelines rather than the comparatively stricter criteria sets of DSM-5-TR, maintains a distinction between substance abuse and dependence, and moves gender incongruence out of its list of mental disorders and into its "Conditions Related to Sexual Health" chapter. Information about ICD-11 can be found at https://icd.who.int/browse11/l-m/en.

Psychodynamic Diagnostic Manual

ICD-11 focuses on diagnoses for public health statistics, whereas the second edition of the *Psychodynamic Diagnostic Manual* (PDM-2) focuses on the psychological health and distress of a particular person. Several psychoanalytical groups worked together to create PDM-2 as a theory-based complement to the descriptive systems of DSM-5-TR and ICD-11. Like DSM-5-TR, PDM-2 includes dimensions that cut across diagnostic categories, along with a thorough account of personality patterns and disorders. PDM-2 includes accounts of the internal experience of a person presenting for treatment (Lingiardi and McWilliams 2017).

Hierarchical Taxonomy of Psychopathology

Like the PDM-2, the Hierarchical Taxonomy of Psychopathology (HiTOP) uses dimensions to cut across DSM-5-TR diagnostic categories. However, the mental health clinicians and researchers working on the HiTOP came from a broad range of theoretical perspectives, not just the psychodynamic community. Their goal was to create a nosology acknowledging that mental health exists along a spectrum between normal and pathological. So instead of a categorical model that declares that a person does or does not have, say, attention-deficit/hyperactivity disorder (ADHD), the HiTOP recognizes that clinical level impairments of attention are related to the fluctuations in attention and activity that everyone experiences. The HiTOP also allows clinicians to diagnose a person across existing diagnostic categories. For example, the HiTOP recognizes the evidence for similarities between ADHD and conduct disorder. Finally, the taxonomy allows for a clinician to see the relationship between a symptom and its constituent components, like maladaptive traits and externalizing behavior. So, instead of simply diagnosing a person with ADHD, a clinician could identify a disinhibited person engaged in antisocial behavior with associated signs, symptoms, and maladaptive behaviors. The HiTOP model is designed to be evidence-based, reliable, and valid, but it is not yet commonly used (Kotov et al. 2017). To get a sense of how it works, a clinician could trial the dimensional model of personality disorders described in Chapter 13, which it resembles.

Power Threat Meaning Framework

The HiTOP, like DSM-5-TR and ICD-11, characterizes the specific mental illness of a particular person. However, no person experiences mental illness or mental health alone. A group of British psychologists, aided by persons with mental illness, recently developed the Power Threat Meaning Framework (PTM) to consider how a person, their family, and their social groups affect the mental health of any particular person. The authors of the PTM observe that in contemporary life, we medicalize most aspects of human distress. We diagnose a person as "depressed" instead of naming the domestic violence or the economic policies they are experiencing as the pathologic state. The PTM reconfigures symptoms as threat responses so that mental distress is, in short, a response to social adversity. The PTM is not a full diagnostic system, but it is a powerful way to engage a person suffering from mental distress. A clinician can incorporate some of the PTM's insights into a diagnostic interview by including four questions (Johnstone et al. 2018, p. 9):

1. What has happened to you? (How is power operating in your life?)
2. How did it affect you? (What kind of threats does this pose?)

3. What sense did you make of it? (What is the meaning of these situations and experiences to you?)
4. What did you have to do to survive? (What kinds of threat responses are you using?)

The PTM also offers questions to help a patient think about their resources and develop their experiences into a narrative, as seen in these two further questions which could be profitably included by a clinician in a diagnostic interview (Johnstone et al. 2018, p. 246):

1. What are your strengths? (What access to power resources do you have?)
2. What is your story? (How does all this fit together?)

As these questions suggest, the PTM provides a thoughtful way to engage the agency of a person experiencing mental distress and to contextualize their experience within their relationships and their narrative understanding of their life.

McHugh's Clusters

Like the PTM's authors, the psychiatrist Paul McHugh developed a different way of thinking about mental illness. Over the past several decades, McHugh argued that by ignoring the putative cause of a disorder, DSM discouraged attempts to understand a disorder (McHugh and Slavney 2012). As an alternative, McHugh proposed grouping mental illnesses into four "clusters" based on the cause of a person's distress. McHugh correlated each cluster with metaphors for treatment. In his first cluster, McHugh (2005) included structural brain diseases that directly disturb psychological functioning. These kinds of disorders can be described as *what disease or condition a person has*. This cluster includes disorders such as Alzheimer's disease, delirium, and schizophrenia. For persons with these illnesses, practitioners seek a cure.

In his second cluster, McHugh included psychological troubles that result from the way someone's mind matured, as in most personality disorders, or roughly who a person *is*. For persons with these illnesses, practitioners act as guides.

In the third cluster, McHugh included disturbances that result from biologically reinforced behaviors such as substance abuse and anorexia nervosa, or what a person *does*. For persons with these illnesses, practitioners attempt to interrupt the behavior.

In the fourth cluster, McHugh included distress due to events that endanger a person's identity, such as bereavement and posttraumatic stress disorder, or what a person *encounters*. For persons with these illnesses, the practitioner helps a person re-script his life story.

McHugh's observations are accessible reading for anyone interested in the meaning of psychiatric diagnosis and classification (McHugh and Slavney 1998) and are useful for a diagnostic interview (Chisolm and Lyketsos 2012). Any clinician can benefit by thinking to themselves, while interviewing a patient:

1. What does this person have?
2. Who is this person?
3. What does this person do that affects their mental health?
4. What has this person encountered that has affected their mental health?

Research Domain Criteria

In its own attempts to pursue the cause of a mental illness, the National Institute of Mental Health (NIMH) is producing the Research Domain Criteria (RDoC) (Insel et al. 2010). At present, RDoC serves as an experimental framework for researching the biological origin of psychiatric illness, but its goal differs from that of DSM-5 (Clark et al. 2017). The ultimate goal of this project is to map behavioral patterns onto etiological cells, genes, molecules, and neural circuits for which new research and new treatments could be developed rather than relying on traditional clinical diagnosis. In this way, a specific behavioral pattern such as impulsivity, which is a trait that may occur in many different current DSM-5-TR diagnoses, might be found through the RDoC to have a relatively unified underlying biological cause (Kozak and Cuthbert 2016). DSM-5-TR takes an important step in the direction of RDoC because it includes dimensions—which are analogous to what the RDoC calls behavioral "domains"—such as impulsivity and negative emotionality, cut across contemporary diagnostic categories, and renews consideration of the etiology of mental distress (Insel and Quirion 2005). The development of RDoC can be followed online (www.nimh.nih.gov/research/research-funded-by-nimh/rdoc/index.shtml).

Rating Scales

Clinicians and researchers have created many rating scales to quantify degrees of health, illness, and impairment. Because the authors of many of these rating scales copyrighted their scales, not all of them are freely available. This poses a special challenge for incorporating validated scales into electronic health records. When possible, a clinician should use a validated scale that they have permission to use. Clinicians may find a good, albeit incomplete, list of rating scales online at www.neurotransmitter.net/ratingscales.html.

References

Aggarwal NK, Lam P, Jiménez-Solomon O, et al: An online training module on the Cultural Formulation Interview: the case of New York State. Psychiatr Serv 69(11):1135–1137, 2018

Aggarwal NK, Cedeno K, Lewis-Fernandez R: Patient and clinician communication practices during the DSM-5 Cultural Formulation Interview field trial. Anthropol Med 27(2):192–211, 2020a

Aggarwal NK, Lam P, Diaz S, et al: Clinician perceptions of implementing the Cultural Formulation Interview on a mixed forensic unit. J Am Acad Psychiatry Law 48(2):216–225, 2020b

Alarcón RD, Frank JB: The Psychotherapy of Hope: The Legacy of Persuasion and Healing. Baltimore, MD, Johns Hopkins University Press, 2011

Allsopp K, Read J, Corcoran R, Kinderman P: Heterogeneity in psychiatric diagnostic classification. Psychiatry Res 279:15–22, 2019

American Psychiatric Association: Diagnostic and Statistical Manual of Mental Disorders, 3rd Edition. Washington, DC, American Psychiatric Association, 1980

American Psychiatric Association: Diagnostic and Statistical Manual of Mental Disorders, 5th Edition. Washington, DC, American Psychiatric Association, 2013

American Psychiatric Association: Diagnostic and Statistical Manual of Mental Disorders, 5th Edition, Text Revision. Washington, DC, American Psychiatric Association, 2022

Aragona M: The concept of mental disorder and the DSM-5. Dialogues in Philosophy, Mental and Neuro Sciences 2:1–14, 2009

Balon R, Beresin EV, Guerrero APS, et al: Clinical skills verification: a problematic examination. Acad Psychiatry 44(3):255–259, 2020

Barroilhet SA, Bieling AE, McCoy TH Jr, Perlis RH: Association between DSM-5 and ICD-11 personality dimensional traits in a general medical cohort and readmission and mortality. Gen Hosp Psychiatry 64:63–67, 2020

Bentall RP: A proposal to classify happiness as a psychiatric disorder. J Med Ethics 18:94–98, 1992

Berganza CE, Mezzich JE: Guía Latinoamericana de Diagnóstico Psiquiátrico. Guadalajara, Jalisco, México, 2004

Bordin ES: The generalizability of the psychoanalytic concept of the working alliance. Psychotherapy (Chic) 16(3):252–260, 1979

Borson S, Scanlan JM, Chen P, Ganguli M: The Mini-Cog as a screen for dementia: validation in a population-based sample. J Am Geriatr Soc 51(10):1451–1454, 2003

Cannon J: Breaking and Mending: A Junior Doctor's Stories of Compassion and Burnout. London, The Borough Press, 2019

263

Carlat DJ: The Psychiatric Interview, 2nd Edition. Philadelphia, PA, Lippincott, Williams & Wilkins, 2005

Case A, Deaton A: Deaths of Despair and the Future of Capitalism. Princeton, NJ, Princeton University Press, 2020

Caspi A, Moffitt TE: All for one and one for all: mental disorders in one dimension. Am J Psychiatry 175(9):831–844, 2018

Caspi A, Houts RM, Ambler A, et al: Longitudinal assessment of mental health disorders and comorbidities across 4 decades among participants in the Dunedin Birth Cohort Study. JAMA Netw Open 3(4):e203221, 2020

Cassell EJ: The Nature of Suffering and the Goals of Medicine. New York, Oxford University Press, 1991

Chekroud AM, Gueorguieva R, Krumholz HM, et al: Reevaluating the efficacy and predictability of antidepressant treatments: a symptom clustering approach. JAMA Psychiatry 74(4):370–378, 2017

Chen YF: Chinese Classification of Mental Disorders (CCMD-3). Psychopathology 35:171–175, 2002

Chisolm MS, Lyketsos CG: Systematic Psychiatric Evaluation: A Step-by-Step Guide to Applying the Perspectives of Psychiatry. Baltimore, MD, Johns Hopkins University Press, 2012

Clark LA, Cuthbert B, Lewis-Fernández R, et al: Three approaches to understanding and classifying mental disorder: ICD-11, DSM-5, and the National Institute of Mental Health's Research Domain Criteria (RDoC). Psychol Sci Public Interest 18(2):72–145, 2017

Cohen H: The nature, methods and purpose of diagnosis. Lancet 241(6227):23–25, 1943

Cole T: Open City. New York, Random House, 2011

Cupitt C: CBT for Psychosis: Process-Orientated Therapies and the Third Wave. New York, Routledge, Taylor & Francis Group, 2019

Davies O: A Theology of Compassion: Metaphysics of Difference and the Renewal of Tradition. Grand Rapids, MI, William B Eerdmans, 2001

Decker HS: The Making of DSM-III: A Diagnostic Manual's Conquest of American Psychiatry. New York, Oxford University Press, 2013

Díaz E, Añez LM, Silva M, et al: Using the Cultural Formulation Interview to build culturally sensitive services. Psychiatr Serv 68(2):112–114, 2017

Digman JM: Personality structure: emergence of the five-factor model. Annu Rev Psychol 41:417–440, 1990

Feinstein AR: Clinical Judgment. Baltimore, MD, Williams & Wilkins, 1967

First MB: DSM-5-TR Handbook of Differential Diagnosis. Washington, DC, American Psychiatric Publishing, 2023

First MB, Bhat V, Adler D, et al: How do clinicians actually use the Diagnostic and Statistical Manual of Mental Disorders in clinical practice and why we need to know more. J Nerv Ment Dis 202(12):841–844, 2014

Fiscella K, Sanders MR: Racial and ethnic disparities in the quality of health care. Annu Rev Public Health 37:375–394, 2016

Flückiger C, Del Re AC, Wampold BE, Horvath AO: The alliance in adult psychotherapy: a meta-analytic synthesis. Psychotherapy (Chic) 55(4):316–340, 2018

Frank JD, Frank JB: Persuasion and Healing: A Comparative Study of Psychotherapy, 3rd Edition. Baltimore, MD, Johns Hopkins University Press, 1991

Gabbard GO, Crisp H: Narcissism and Its Discontents: Diagnostic Dilemmas and Treatment Strategies With Narcissistic Patients. Washington, DC, American Psychiatric Association Publishing, 2018

Grisanzio KA, Goldstein-Piekarski AN, Wang MY, et al: Transdiagnostic symptom clusters and associations with brain, behavior, and daily function in mood, anxiety, and trauma disorders. JAMA Psychiatry 75(2):201–209, 2018

Grob GN: Origins of DSM-I: a study in appearance and reality. Am J Psychiatry 148:421–431, 1991

Hayes SC, Hofmann SG (eds): Beyond the DSM: Toward a Process-Based Alternative for Diagnosis and Mental Health Treatment. Oakland, CA, Context Press, 2020

Hilt RJ, Nussbaum AM: DSM-5 Pocket Guide for Child and Adolescent Mental Health. Arlington, VA, American Psychiatric Association Publishing, 2016

Hirota H: Expelling the Poor: Atlantic Seaboard States and the Nineteenth-Century Origins of American Immigration Policy. New York, Oxford University Press, 2017

Houts AC: Fifty years of psychiatric nomenclature: reflections on the 1943 War Department Technical Bulletin, Medical 203. J Clin Psychol 56:935–967, 2000

Huang K, Yeomans M, Brooks AW, et al: It doesn't hurt to ask: question-asking increases liking. J Pers Soc Psychol 113(3):430–452, 2017

Hunter KM: How Doctors Think: Clinical Judgment and the Practice of Medicine. New York, Oxford University Press, 2005

Ingram SH, South SC: The longitudinal impact of DSM-5 Section III specific personality disorders on relationship satisfaction. Pers Disord 12(2):140–149, 2021

Inouye SK, van Dyck CH, Alessi CA, et al: Clarifying confusion: the confusion assessment method. A new method for detection of delirium. Ann Intern Med 113(12):941–948, 1990

Insel T, Quirion R: Psychiatry as a clinical neuroscience discipline. JAMA 294:2221–2224, 2005

Insel T, Cuthbert B, Garvey M, et al: Research Domain Criteria (RDoC): toward a new classification framework for research on mental disorders. Am J Psychiatry 167:748–751, 2010

Jarvis GE, Kirmayer LJ, Gómez-Carrillo A, et al: Update on the Cultural Formulation Interview. Focus Am Psychiatr Publ 18(1):40–46, 2020

Jibson MD, Broquet KE, Anzia JM, et al; ABPN Task Force on Clinical Skills Verification Rater Training: Clinical skills verification in general psychiatry: recommendations of the ABPN Task Force on Rater Training. Acad Psychiatry 36(5):363–368, 2012

Johnson RL, Sadosty AT, Weaver AL, et al: To sit or not to sit? Ann Emerg Med 51:188–193, 2008

Johnstone L, Boyle M, Cromby J, et al: The Power Threat Meaning Framework: Towards the Identification of Patterns in Emotional Distress, Unusual Experiences and Troubled or Troubling Behaviour, as an Alternative to Functional Psychiatric Diagnosis. Leicester, UK, British Psychological Society, 2018

Juul D, Brooks BA, Jozefowicz R, et al: Clinical skills assessment: the effects of moving certification requirements into neurology, child neurology, and psychiatric residency training. J Grad Med Educ 7(1):98–100, 2015

Kendell R, Jablensky A: Distinguishing between the validity and utility of psychiatric diagnoses. Am J Psychiatry 160:4–12, 2003

Kendler KS: The dappled nature of causes of psychiatric illness: replacing the organic-functional/hardware-software dichotomy with empirically based pluralism. Mol Psychiatry 17:377–388, 2012

Kendler KS: The structure of psychiatric science. Am J Psychiatry 171(9):931–938, 2014a

Kendler KS: DSM issues: incorporation of biological tests, avoidance of reification, and an approach to the "box canyon problem." Am J Psychiatry 171(12):1248–1250, 2014b

Kendler KS: The phenomenology of major depression and the representativeness and nature of DSM criteria. Am J Psychiatry 173(8):771–780, 2016

Kernberg OF: Severe Personality Disorders. New Haven, CT, Yale University Press, 1984

Keshavarzi H, Khan F, Alu B, Awaad R: Applying Islamic Principles to Clinical Mental Health Care. New York, Routledge, 2020

King LS: Medical Thinking: A Historical Preface. Princeton, NJ, Princeton University Press, 1982

Kinghorn WA: Whose disorder? A constructive MacIntyrean critique of psychiatric nosology. J Med Philos 36:187–205, 2011

Kinghorn WA, Nussbaum AM: Prescribing Together: A Relational Guide to Psychopharmacology. Washington, DC, American Psychiatric Association Press, 2021

Kleinman A, Eisenberg L, Good B: Culture, illness, and care: critical lessons from anthropologic and cross-cultural research. Ann Intern Med 88:251–258, 1978

Konecky B, Meyer EC, Marx BP, et al: Using the WHODAS 2.0 to assess functional disability associated with DSM-5 mental disorders. Am J Psychiatry 171(8):818–820, 2014

Kotov R, Krueger RF, Watson D, et al: The Hierarchical Taxonomy of Psychopathology (HiTOP): A dimensional alternative to traditional nosologies. J Abnorm Psychol 126(4):454–477, 2017

Kozak MJ, Cuthbert BN: The NIMH Research Domain Criteria Initiative: background, issues, and pragmatics. Psychophysiology 53(3):286–297, 2016

Kupfer DJ, Regier DA: Neuroscience, clinical evidence, and the future of psychiatric classification in DSM-5. Am J Psychiatry 168:672–674, 2011

Lewis-Fernández R, Hinton DE, Laria AJ: Culture and the anxiety disorders: recommendations for DSM-5. Depress Anxiety 27:212–229, 2010

Lewis-Fernández R, Aggarwal NK, Hinton L, et al: DSM-5 Handbook on the Cultural Formulation Interview. Washington, DC, American Psychiatric Publishing, 2016

Lingiardi V, McWilliams N: Psychodynamic Diagnostic Manual: PDM-2, 2nd Edition. New York, Guilford, 2017

Little M: Talking cure and curing talk. J R Soc Med 98:210–212, 2005

Lizardi D, Oquendo MA, Graver R: Clinical pitfalls in the diagnosis of ataque de nervios: a case study. Transcult Psychiatry 46:463–486, 2009

MacIntyre AC: Dependent Rational Animals: Why Human Beings Need the Virtues. Chicago, IL, Open Court Publishing, 2012

MacKinnon RA, Michels R, Buckley PJ: The Psychiatric Interview in Clinical Practice, 2nd Edition. Washington, DC, American Psychiatric Publishing, 2006

MacKinnon RA, Michels R, Buckley PJ: The Psychiatric Interview in Clinical Practice, 3rd Edition. Washington, DC, American Psychiatric Publishing, 2016

McHugh PR: Striving for coherence: psychiatry's efforts over classification. JAMA 293:2526–2528, 2005

McHugh P: Review of "The Loss of Sadness: How Psychiatry Transformed Normal Sorrow Into Depressive Disorder." N Engl J Med 357:947–948, 2007

McHugh P, Slavney PR: The Perspectives of Psychiatry, 2nd Edition. Baltimore, MD, Johns Hopkins University Press, 1998

McHugh P, Slavney PR: Mental illness—comprehensive evaluation or checklist? N Engl J Med 366:1853–1855, 2012

Metzl J: The Protest Psychosis: How Schizophrenia Became a Black Disease. Boston, MA, Beacon Press, 2009

Milinkovic MS, Tiliopoulos N: A systematic review of the clinical utility of the DSM-5 section III alternative model of personality disorder. Pers Disord 11(6):377–397, 2020

Mills S, Wolitzky-Taylor K, Xiao AQ, et al: Training on the DSM-5 Cultural Formulation Interview improves cultural competence in general psychiatry residents: a multi-site study. Acad Psychiatry 40(5):829–834, 2016

Morrison J, Muñoz RA: Boarding Time: The Psychiatry Candidate's New Guide to Part II of the ABPN Examination. Washington, DC, American Psychiatric Publishing, 2009

Mundt C, Backenstrass M: Psychotherapy and classification: psychological, psychodynamic, and cognitive aspects. Psychopathology 38:219–222, 2005

Nakane Y, Nakane H: Classification systems for psychiatric diseases currently used in Japan. Psychopathology 35:191–194, 2002

Neugeboren J, Sederer LI, Friedman MB: The Diagnostic Manual of Mishegas: DMOM. CreateSpace Independent Publishing Platform, 2013

Newton-Howes G, Clark LA, Chanen A: Personality disorder across the life course. Lancet 385(9969):727–734, 2015

Nussbaum AM: Alternatives to war within medicine: from conscientious objection to nonviolent conflict about contested medical practices. Perspect Biol Med 62(3):434–451, 2019 31495790

Oberlander J: The Social Medicine Reader, 3rd Edition. Durham, NC, Duke University Press, 2019

Otero-Ojeda AA: Third Cuban Glossary of Psychiatry (GC-3): key features and contributions. Psychopathology 35:181–184, 2002

Parsons T: Illness and the role of the physician: a sociological perspective. Am J Orthopsychiatry 21:452–460, 1951

Pétrement S: Simone Weil: A Life. New York, Pantheon Books, 1976

Pierre J: The borders of mental disorders in psychiatry and the DSM: past, present, and future. J Psychiatr Pract 16:375–386, 2010

Pinto RZ, Ferreira ML, Oliveira VC, et al: Patient-centred communication is associated with positive therapeutic alliance: a systematic review. J Physiother 58(2):77–87, 2012

Radden J, Sadler JZ: The Virtuous Psychiatrist: Character Ethics in Psychiatric Practice. New York, Oxford University Press, 2010

Rao NR, Kodali R, Mian A, et al: Psychiatric residents' attitudes toward and experiences with the clinical-skills verification process: a pilot study on U.S. and international medical graduates. Acad Psychiatry 36(4):316–322, 2012

Raskin JD: What might an alternative to the DSM suitable for psychotherapists look like? J Humanist Psychol 59(3):368–375, 2019

Regier DA: Dimensional approaches to psychiatric classification: refining the research agenda for DSM-5: an introduction. Int J Methods Psychiatr Res 16(suppl 1):1–5, 2007

Regier DA, Narrow WE, Kuhl EA, et al: The conceptual development of DSM-5. Am J Psychiatry 166:645–650, 2009

Reichenberg LW, Seligman L: Selecting Effective Treatments, 5th Edition. New York, Wiley, 2016

Roberts LW: A Clinical Guide to Psychiatric Ethics. Washington, DC, American Psychiatric Association Publishing, 2016

Robertson K: Active listening: more than just paying attention. Aust Fam Physician 34:1053–1055, 2005

Rüsch N, Angermeyer MC, Corrigan PW: Mental illness stigma: concepts, consequences, and initiatives to reduce stigmas. Eur Psychiatry 20:529–539, 2005

Sachdev P: Schizophrenia-like psychosis and epilepsy: the status of the association. Am J Psychiatry 155(3):325–336, 1998

Saini V, Garcia-Armesto S, Klemperer D, et al: Drivers of poor medical care. Lancet 390(10090):178–190, 2017

Shahrokh NC, Hales RE, Phillips KA, et al: The Language of Mental Health: A Glossary of Psychiatric Terms. Washington, DC, American Psychiatric Publishing, 2011

Shea SC: Psychiatric Interviewing: The Art of Understanding, 2nd Edition. Philadelphia, PA, WB Saunders, 1998

Shea SC: Psychiatric Interviewing: The Art of Understanding, 3rd Edition. Edinburgh, Elsevier, 2017

Shweder RA: Why Do Men Barbecue? Recipes for Cultural Psychology. Cambridge, MA, Harvard University Press, 2003

Simpson SA, McDowell AK: The Clinical Interview: Skills for More Effective Patient Encounters. New York, Routledge, 2019

Skodol AE, Morey LC, Bender DS, Oldham JM: The Alternative DSM-5 Model for Personality Disorders: a clinical application. Am J Psychiatry 172(7):606–613, 2015

Stein DJ, Phillips KA, Bolton D, et al: What is a mental/psychiatric disorder? From DSM-IV to DSM-V. Psychol Med 40(11):1759–1765, 2010

Sullivan HS: The Collected Works of Harry Stack Sullivan, Vol 1: The Psychiatric Interview. Edited by Perry HS, Gawel ML. New York, WW Norton, 1954

Summers RF, Barber JP: Therapeutic alliance as a measurable psychotherapy skill. Acad Psychiatry 27:160–165, 2003

Swayden KJ, Anderson KK, Connelly LM, et al: Effect of sitting vs. standing on perception of provider time at bedside: a pilot study. Patient Educ Couns 86(2):166–171, 2012

Totura CMW, Fields SA, Karver MS: The role of the therapeutic relationship in psychopharmacological treatment outcomes: a meta-analytic review. Psychiatr Serv 69(1):41–47, 2018

Tremain H, McEnery C, Fletcher K, Murray G: The therapeutic alliance in digital mental health interventions for serious mental illnesses: narrative review. JMIR Ment Health 7(8):e17204, 2020

Tsoi KKF, Chan JYC, Hirai HW, et al: Cognitive tests to detect dementia: a systematic review and meta-analysis. JAMA Intern Med 175(9):1450–1458, 2015

VanderWeele TJ: Activities for flourishing: an evidence-based guide. Journal of Positive School Psychology 4(1):79–91, 2020

Wallace ER: Psychiatry and its nosology: a historico-philosophical overview, in Philosophical Perspective on Psychiatric Diagnostic Classification. Edited by Sadler JZ, Wiggins OP, Schwartz MA. Baltimore, MD, Johns Hopkins University Press, 1994, pp 16–88

Wang S, Nussbaum AM: DSM-5 Pocket Guide for Elder Mental Health. Arlington, VA, American Psychiatric Association Publishing, 2017

Weekers LC, Hutsebaut J, Bach B, Kamphuis JH: Scripting the DSM-5 Alternative Model for Personality Disorders assessment procedure: a clinically feasible multi-informant multi-method approach. Pers Ment Health 14(3):304–318, 2020

Weiden PJ: Understanding and addressing adherence issues in schizophrenia: from theory to practice. J Clin Psychiatry 68(suppl 14):14–19, 2007

Wilson M: DSM-III and the transformation of American psychiatry: a history. Am J Psychiatry 150:399–410, 1993

World Health Organization: Measuring Health and Disability: Manual for WHO Disability Assessment Schedule (WHODAS 2.0). Edited by Üstün TB, Kostanjsek N, Chatterji S, et al. Geneva, World Health Organization, 2010

Yager J: Specific components of bedside manner in the general hospital psychiatric consultation: 12 concrete suggestions. Psychosomatics 30:209–212, 1989

Zimmerman M: Interview Guide for Evaluating DSM-IV Psychiatric Disorders and the Mental Status Examination. East Greenwich, RI, Psych Products Press, 1994

Zulman DM, Haverfield MC, Shaw JG, et al: Practices to foster physician presence and connection with patients in the clinical encounter. JAMA 323(1):70–81, 2020

Index

*Page numbers printed in **boldface** type refer to tables.*

271

Behavior (*continued*)
  nonverbal communicative
      behaviors, 74
  socially deviant, 11
  suicidal, **183**
Bentall, Richard, 7
Bereavement, 55. *See also* Death;
    Grief
Binge eating, 111. *See also*
    Feeding and eating
    disorders
Bipolar and related disorders, in
    DSM-5-TR, 83–87, **198**
Bipolar I disorder, in DSM-5-TR,
    83–85, **198**
Bipolar II disorder, in
    DSM-5-TR, 85–87, **198**
Blame, 101
BMI, 110. *See also* Feeding and
    eating disorders
Board certification.
    See American Board of
    Psychiatry and Neurology
    (ABPN), clinical skills
    evaluation
Borderline personality disorder
    dimensional diagnosis of,
        243–245
    in DSM-5-TR, 174
Bordin, Edward, 15

Caffeine intoxication, in
    DSM-5-TR, 138
Caffeine withdrawal, in
    DSM-5-TR, 139
Cannabis intoxication, in
    DSM-5-TR, 141
Cannabis use disorder, in
    DSM-5-TR, 139–141
Cannabis withdrawal, in
    DSM-5-TR, 141–142
Cannon, Joanna, 25
Caregiver, goals of, 217–219,
    219–220

Case examples
  of death, 54–55
  of major depressive disorder,
      54–55
  of neurocognitive disorder,
      56–59
  of personality disorder, 59–60
  of schizophrenia, 51–52
Catatonic behavior, 80
Categorical models, 6–7, 50, 60
Child abuse. *See* Psychosocial
    functioning
Children. *See also* Adolescents
  child maltreatment and
      neglect problems,
      183–186
  gender dysphoria in
      DSM-5-TR, 127–128
Clinical skills evaluations
    (CSEs), 221–223
Clinician-Rated Dimensions of
    Psychosis Symptom
    Severity, 227, **228–230**
Clumsiness, 76
Cognition. *See also* Memories;
    Neurocognitive disorders
  mental status examination
      during, 213
Cognitive-behavioral therapy,
    therapeutic alliance and,
    15–16
Cohen, Henry, 5
Communication. *See also*
    Therapeutic alliance
  with patient, 22
Communication disorder, 73
Compulsions, 31. *See also*
    Obsessions
Conduct disorder, in DSM-5-TR,
    130–134
Confidentiality, 22
Counseling, **191**
Cultural explanation of
    perceived cause, 47